THE WAY TO LIVE IN HEALTH AND PHYSICAL FITNESS
(ORIGINAL VERSION, RESTORED)

By GEORGE HACKENSCHMIDT

Originally Published in 1908

PUBLISHED BY O'Faolain Patriot LLC, Copyright 2011
info@PhysicalCultureBooks.com
Published in the United States of America

ISBN-13: 978-1466466302

ISBN-10: 1466466308

To Order More Copies Visit: Physical Culture Books.com

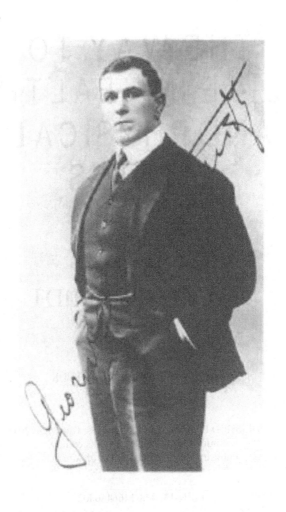

The information contained in this publication is for historical and educational purposes only and is not designed to and does not provide medical, nutritional, or health advice, diagnosis, or opinion for any health or individual problem. The material presented is not a substitute for medical or other professional health services from a qualified health care provider who is familiar with the unique facts of the individual, and should not be used in place of a visit, call, consultation, or advice of a physician or other healthcare provider. Individuals should always consult a qualified health care provider about any health concern and prior to undertaking any new treatment. The publisher assumes no responsibility and specifically disclaims all liability for any consequence relating directly or indirectly to any action or inaction that a reader takes based on any information contained herein.

Be advised that no one should undertake exercises in the nature of those addressed in this book without prior consultation with a physician. Nor does the publisher make any representations concerning whether any of the exercises or suggestions provided by the trainers or physical fitness specialists featured in this book would be effective or appropriate for the reader's needs or expectations. The publisher expressly disclaims any and all responsibility and/or liabilities that might result from the uninformed or misinformed application of the techniques identified herein as well as for any unsupervised physical fitness training.

Finally, the publisher disclaims any and all liabilities arising from the use of any equipment featured in this book and makes no representations as to the utility, safety, or adequacy of the equipment generally or with respect to any specific purpose.

TABLE OF CONTENTS

I. INTRODUCTION	p.8
II. WHY SHOULD WE BE STRONG?	p.14
III. ADAPTABILITY AND CHARACTERISTICS	p.21
IV. PHYSICAL PERFECTION AND STRENGTH	p.27
V. NUTRITION	p.39
VI. REST AND WHOLESOME SOUP	p.46
VII. TRAINING	p.49
VIII. EXERCISES WITHOUT WEIGHTS	p.55
IX. MUSCLE EXERCISES WITH WEIGHTS	p.70
X. WEIGHTS FOR EXERCISES	p.88
XI. EXERCISES FOR ATHLETES	p.91
XII. TIME TABLES FOR TRAINING	p.110
XIII. DR. VON KRAJEWSKI, THE FATHER OF ATHLETICS AND HIS SYSTEM OF LIFE	p.115
The Story of my Life	p.122

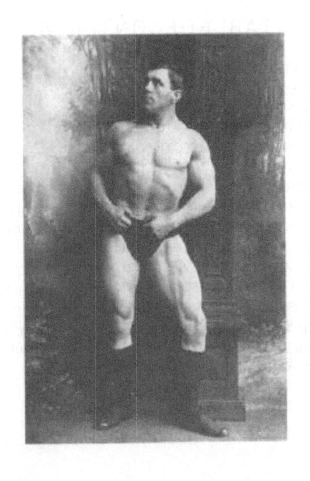

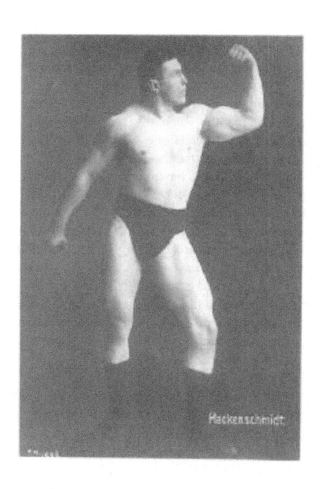

I
INTRODUCTION

IT is not at all improbable that many persons will raise objections to the title of this book, on the grounds that the Road of Life, which I may point out, is by no means one which the average person would wish to tread. These will very probably suggest (without having troubled to read these pages) that they have no desire to distinguish themselves either as wrestlers or as weight-lifters, and that in consequence Hackenschmidt's Way of Life must necessarily diverge pretty considerably from theirs.

But, as will be seen, it has not been my design to confine myself to laying down a series of rules for strong men and athletes only: my object in writing this book has been rather to lay before my readers such data as may enable them to secure Health as well as Strength.

It is true that a large section is devoted to exercises, etc., which will tend to the development of Strength, but then, surely, it is the desire of every man to increase his physical powers. Health can never be divorced from Strength. The second is an inevitable sequel to the first. A man can only fortify himself against disease by strengthening his body in such manner as will enable it to defy the attacks of any malady.

The progress of civilization has been chiefly marked by the progress of Medical Science. The study and practice of Surgery and Medicine have grown amazingly during the past few generations. Sanitary arrangements have been almost perfected, while the precautions and safeguards against disease, which have been instituted by states and municipalities, are simply admirable.

Despite all these improvements, one can scarcely come across any official health report which does not bewail an all-round degeneration of physique.

There are fewer plagues and pestilences, but there would appear to be an infinitely greater number of sickly, weedy, stunted people than there used to be.

The reason is not far to seek. There is an universal urban immigration, a vast increase in the numbers of those who are engaged in indoor and sedentary occupation, and only here and there is any attempt made to combat the consequent unhealthy conditions of life with the only satisfactory weapon, Rational Physical Exercise.

Unfortunately, the majority of people seem to associate the words Physical Culture with huge muscular development. Men who do not entertain any ambition of figuring as professional athletes consequently omit to pay any attention to the care of their bodies.

They do not wish to be ill, but they nevertheless appear to consider that occasional ill-health is the inevitable fate of every son of Adam and must be endured, if not exactly welcomed.

Now, apart from extraordinary causes, there is absolutely no reason why any man should ever be ill, as long as he keeps his body so physically fit as to safeguard it against any breakdown. Fifteen or twenty minutes' daily exercise will be all sufficient for this purpose. Surely no very heavy price to pay for such a valuable result.

This is no idle, unfounded claim. Any reader who may fancy it to be such, need but make say a fortnight's experiment of the course prescribed. Even before that period expired, the beneficial result would be readily- perceived.

The exercise, however, must be rational, suitable exercise. Movements such as will tune up the whole frame and keep every organ and muscle working harmoniously together.

I do not claim to be the first preacher of this gospel, nor could I venture to pose as such, seeing the vast library of books, which have been published from time to time, on this subject of Physical Culture and its advantages. But from a more or less complete study of the said works I have come to the conclusion that the vast majority of them, or at all events of the most instructive ones, have been so written as to be largely unintelligible to " the man in the street," while others, and these, unfortunately, by no means the least popular, deal almost exclusively with systems of exercise which their authors have never practised themselves, nor which, to my knowledge, have ever been practised by any really strong man.

I have, therefore, confined myself to dealing only with such systems of exercise, diet, rest, etc., as my own observation and experience have shown thoroughly sound and reliable, proved to be such in numberless instances, and in describing them have sought to set down my views in such language as will be readily comprehended by every reader, avoiding as far as possible all unnecessary technical details. Whether I have failed or succeeded in these endeavors remains for my readers to judge.

EXERCISES FOR YOUNG AND OLD

There is one point on which I would wish to lay stress, and that is, that no matter what age a man may have attained, he is by no means too old to commence exercise. I have devoted several pages to exercises with heavy weights, for the purpose of developing Strength (with a capital S), and I sincerely hope that none of my readers will be frightened on this account.

It may be suggested that there is no reason why a man should go to the trouble and exertion of struggling with heavy weights, since there is no crying necessity for that particular man to acquire any phenomenal degree of strength.

To that I would reply by asking why a man should desire to be weak?

He was endowed by his Creator with muscles and sinews which would enable him to cope successfully with such physical feats as he might be faced with during his earthly career.

Modern social conditions have deprived him of that open-air life and hard physical exertion which would have kept these muscles and sinews in good condition and sound working order.

But since he has been separated from the natural physical advantages, which were freely offered to him in bygone centuries, he should surely avail himself of the efficient substitutes which are offered to him by trained and practised physical culturists and the method of which I have here endeavored to set forth.

For it is only by exercising with heavy weights that any man can hope to develop really great strength. He should of course combine these exercises with skipping, running jumping and gymnastics of every description in order to similarly develop his activity and agility, but unless he sedulously carries out the bar-bell and dumb-bell exercises as well he can never acquire really great physical powers.

The man of forty or fifty, however, who has passed the age when the desire for great strength is still active and who only desires the acquisition and preservation of health may content himself with the exercises designed solely for that end.

But I would strongly urge on all such, that it is their bounden duty to encourage, by every means in their power, the pursuit of Strength among all the youths of their district. Persuade the boys and young men in every locality to band themselves together for the purpose of forming Physical Culture Clubs and Gymnasia, where they can exercise and develop their bodies.

Enthusiasm will soon be evoked. The public-houses and other even less desirable resorts will suffer (no bad result this), the country and the human race will benefit; nor will the minds of the youths in question lack a sympathetic development.

The old notion that physical prowess was inseparable from a dull intelligence is completely exploded, and happily so, seeing that it was about the most harmful notion which has ever been entertained by man. A boy whose attention is directed to physical exercise will speedily recognize its benefits and healthful pleasures, and will consequently readily and instinctively avoid all harmful excesses. He will also inevitably develop an interest in his own anatomy and thereby in what are now known as " the mysteries of life "; soon, it is to be hoped (by the spread of Physical Culture), to become less mysterious than they have been hitherto.

II
WHY SHOULD WE BE STRONG?

IT is a well-known fact that the majority of men today are relatively weak, whereas the struggle for existence demands now more than at any previous epoch that we should all be strong!

The reader may think that physical strength is not a necessity, but I will try and prove to him that man cannot derive real enjoyment from life unless he possesses a powerful and healthy physical constitution. A famous physician expressed himself as follows: " If I think of my experiences during a thirty years' practice, I cannot recall many cases where a patient became ill through too great an exertion on his physical system, whereas I remember many hundreds who have contracted serious illness through mental strain and brain fag, and their complete recovery invariably was a slow and difficult process.

" I have come to the distinct conclusion, that the physical constitution of the human frame never was intended merely for study, but rather for manual and bodily exercise. I have found that those who have lived an active outdoor life have retained and enjoyed a brightness born of health far longer than others. Such people always enjoyed their meals, seldom suffered from indigestion, headaches, or nervous exhaustion. Indigestion is the direct result of the ineffective performance by the digestive organs of their functions, brought on either, on the one hand, by over-eating or consuming unsuitable food and noxious drugs, or, on the other hand, by physical inactivity. What a contrast to these are the constitutions of those people who toil in rooms or do mental work only; they often suffer from heat in the head, cold feet, sluggish digestion, or weak and inactive bowels. Few among them are those who do not suffer from some form of nervous complaint. The feeling of comfort and happiness is almost unknown to them.

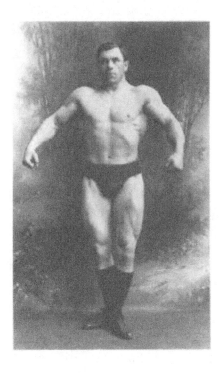

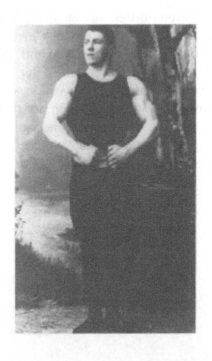

" We know that every organ, when actively performing its duties, demands a rich supply of blood; its veins become enlarged, and, considering the fact that much more blood flows through a muscle while it is in activity than while it is at rest, it is evident that the same rule holds good as regards the brain. If more blood flows to the brain than under normal conditions, the other parts of the body are more or less depleted of it, feet and arms become cold, and the feeling is, to say the least, uncomfortable. I have the firm conviction that in time everyone will recognize the necessity of daily bodily exercises in one form or another, as an ordinary counterpart to one's daily mental exertions."

Human life is not unlike a commercial business establishment. There is a continual exchange of matter, and just as the commercial establishment suffers and decays when the turnover diminishes, or the stock of goods accumulates without being disposed of, so a continuous exchange of matter is needful for our body, if a paralysis in life's activity—in another word, illness—is to be averted or a complete stoppage—that is death—prevented. Just as a commercial business flourishes the more this interchange of goods takes place, so a man benefits in health and comfort and can get out of himself better service in any useful direction, if the exchange of matter in his body takes place regularly and frequently.

In life, however, cause and effect continually change their role. As the man of commerce must not be idle, but must be active from early morn till night, so we can only keep our wonderful organism in constant regularity by repeated impulse to, and continual exertion in, its respective functions. This is the only way to prevent exhaustion of the organs and to contribute properly to their strengthening, improvement, and preservation. You will ask how far we can attain this, and how it is possible to effect such a deep influence on a whole life's activity. I would reply to this in the following manner:

Every movement is produced by the muscles. These are skeins of flesh tissues, which have the vital faculty of contraction and extension. They are attached by sinews to the foundation of bone, and by contraction they change in position or alter in shape. The impulse to this movement is carried by the nerves, which have their centre in the brain. The nerves are not unlike the metal wires of a battery, which carry the electricity whither it is needed, and in like manner the brain sends the impulse by means of the nerves to whatever muscles it wills. If, therefore, the muscles are frequently set in motion by our will, they are first of all strengthened in their power of contraction and of executing different movements; and are thus brought to their full development and perfection.

Those muscles which are left inactive to a greater or lesser extent lose their power of contraction and naturally deteriorate. This retrogression appears in the shape of muscular weakness and exhaustion. We find these effects mostly among people of the so-called upper classes. They are tired by the least exertion, are afraid of the slightest draught, and are often martyrs to weak nerves, rheumatism, and catarrh. Ladies who take no regular physical exercise, or who are not engaged in any occupation entailing such, are invariably startled and frightened by the least unexpected noise, such as the sudden opening of a door. They become "nervous" and often hysterically affected by unlooked-for occurrences of even the most paltry nature. Now all these ills and disorders are unknown to those who take regular physical exercise, for by it their nervous system obtains strength and firmness and that endurance which is the essence of a good constitution.

Through the pressure of blood and the accumulation of nerve fluid in the brain, the nervous man is filled with continual anxiety for his physical well being. His overstrung nerves cause him to imagine all kinds of ailments. One thought after another flits across his mind; at one time he believes himself to be strong, at another weak, now he fancies himself well, now ill. He is tormented by a never-ending strife between hope of life and fear of death. Hope after hope slips successively from his grasp, and finally he sinks into a more or less dangerous mental illness, the result of which may easily lead him to seek release in self-destruction.

The most effectual means of preventing all the disadvantages and evil consequences of a neglected exercise of body and muscles is methodical physical training.

Just as the man of sedentary habits and weak body possesses a correspondingly sluggish mind and lack of energy, so he who assiduously pursues a physical development gains not only that desired government of his organs, but in marked degree obtains a thorough mastery of his will and, consequently, an easy and contented mind.

The frequent employment of one's will power masters all organs of movement and trains them to perform feats which otherwise would have been difficult, painful, and even impossible. The man becomes independent and self-reliant ; he will never be a coward, and, when real danger threatens, he is the one who is looked up to by others. The knowledge of one's strength entails a real mastery over oneself; it breeds energy and courage, helps one over the most difficult tasks of life, and procures contentment and true enjoyment of living. Who would still lag behind in inactivity and weakness?

III
ADAPTABILITY AND CHARACTERISTICS

I SHOULD like to say a few words upon this subject, and I know that I echo the opinions of well-known authorities on training.

It is natural that a sound constitution, inherited from healthy parents, and a proportionate build, should be great advantages for a future athlete. Especially should the heart and the lungs be normal, although I quite admit that one finds strong and healthy children of comparatively weak parents, and vice versa; and I know of many cases in which seemingly weak or ailing youngsters have developed into strong men, thanks to their energetic endurance and steadfast desire to achieve that result.

As regards stature, I will only mention that a moderate height of from 5 ft 6 in. to 6 ft seems very favorable, seeing that that is the average of most strong men (I myself am 5 ft 9½ in.); but, of course, there are exceptions to this. The body should be built very uniformly, so that the whole appearance makes a harmonious impression. It would not matter much whether the arms or legs were somewhat under the normal length, but a short trunk would indicate a poor development of the important inner organs, such as lungs, heart, and stomach, and, therefore, would be less favorable. For wrestling and boxing, long arms are an advantage, whilst for weight-lifting I should prefer shorter arms, but, of course, the principal point lies with the more or less favorable leverage capacity of the frame. Now it is a fact that by reasonable physical exercise the growth of the structure is encouraged; by reasonable exercise I mean such as is adapted to the personal constitution and the age of the individual.

During the process of growth and bodily development, say until about the twenty-fifth year, one ought not to practise any extreme athletic feats, but ought to pay chief attention to agility and alertness. Great exertions in youth hinder the growth and bring a too early maturity, which tends to shorten life.

For great feats of strength with heavy weights experience teaches, that between the years of thirty and forty is the most favorable age; I suppose though, that I am an exception, as I had already established world's records before I was twenty-one.

It will, however, I think, be of interest to quote the opinions of a few eminent authorities on these subjects.

ADOLPH ANDRUSCHKEWITZSCH, who is a well-known Russian athlete and authority on Physical Culture, of Reval, says:—

"Every country can produce strong men; Estland (Russia) in general offers no special advantages, although one might argue that Estland, similarly to, perhaps, Eastern Prussia (the native country of Sandow, Sturm, and Siegfried), has few industries, and that therefore its inhabitants pursue their vocations principally in the open, breathe pure air, and live on healthy, unadulterated foods. Estland's percentage of people of consumptive tendencies is very low, just as is that of Eastern Prussia; while in the thickly-populated kingdom of Saxony the ravages of this terrible disease are very severe. At the same time, however, Arthur Saxon, who is undoubtedly the best weight-lifter of the present time, hails from Saxony!

" To become a good athlete the candidate should, in my opinion, be possessed of a strong boned frame and a good sound chest, and he should be generally healthy. To attain this, he ought to avoid worry and strenuous daily toil; the choice of food is of secondary consideration, as long as his meals are wholesome, regular, and properly digested. Alcohols and stimulants may produce seeming momentary strength, but in reality they weaken the system.

" An essential point is, that the candidate puts his life and soul into the study of proper training; enduring will power is the mightiest factor for good results, and for the production of men like Hackenschmidt, Lurich, Sandow, Saxon, Aberg, or Hoeppener."

MAX DANTHAGE, of Vienna, the well-known athlete- gymnast, says:—

" My principal nourishment consists of meat. I drink very little. For my breakfast I take very weak tea and a buttered roll. With my luncheon and dinner about one pint of light beer; I never drink wines, spirits or water. Except in summer, I do not bathe often, but I wash and take douches frequently, and use the towel well. I never fail to go through this washing performance after every exertion which has produced perspiration, and I may add that

I use cold water. This cold washing should, however, not be of longer duration than a few seconds, if the body has been perspiring. As regards training, I recommend the following items:— "Moderation in everything, of whatever nature. " Daily short baths and vigorous rubbing down.

Daily physical exercise, avoiding great feats of strength but performing feats of endurance, and this until one begins to perspire slightly.

" I began to practise physical exercises regularly and systematically six years ago, when I was thirty-one. Of course, I went through the usual physical training at school, between the years of six and seventeen, and after this I continued gymnastics a few times per week on the horizontal bar at home in the garden and practised with small dumb-bells. I like swimming, and have always indulged in this pleasurable exercise when I had an opportunity. Skating and cycling were other hobbies, and anything appertaining to gymnastical sports, except fencing and riding. I have never made a study of any particular line of sport. My present endeavor is to develop my body in every direction, and so give it every day not only its necessary food, but also to exercise it until, as I said before, my pores open and perspiration commences. The precise observation of all these points fitted me for such feats of endurance as you are familiar with, and my hardihood has become proverbial among my friends and acquaintances. I have been called the man who never catches cold or catarrh, and who is never ill. My measurements are: Height, 5 ft 8 in.; chest, deflated, 36½ in., normal, 37½ in., inflated, 40¾ in.; thighs, 24¼ in. ; calves, 15 in.; biceps, 14¾ in.; wrist, 7¼ in.; weight, 159 lb."

* * * * *

I must draw the reader's attention to the fact that Danthage, who is a member of the Royal Opera Band, is the gymnast who, among other feats of endurance, made what the Germans call the deep knee-bend 6,000 times during four consecutive hours. The " knee-bend " is a capital exercise, and consists in bending your knees outwards by moving from the erect position to a sort of sitting posture without moving the feet.

Monsieur GASNIER, the well-known athlete of Barnum and Bailey's Circus, writes:—

" Lots of people ask me whether they can become strong. Most certainly! You all can acquire great strength, if you have the will and proper guidance. But before all you must cultivate will power, and this first lesson is the most important one. If physical exercises alone, without your will and mind, were all that was needful, every one could become a strong man, whether he be a brain or muscle worker.

" The laborer, however, who never particularly uses his mind while he strains all his muscles in hard toil, and every day lifts weights, does not necessarily augment his strength.

" Those who would like to have well-developed muscles should guard against over-exertion and impetuous exercise. One can become strong by daily exercises with light dumb-bells, and such exercises should take place either two hours before or after meals. Before one begins with heavier weights, one ought to study what weights would not cause over-exertion for the constitution as it then is.

" I recommend cold baths twice a week, or dail y cold washing of the whole body with a sponge, and this immediately upon rising in the morning. This is very healthy and invigorating.

" I should advise an amateur to vary the duration of his exercises; for instance, if he feels particularly fit he may exercise a little longer than on days when he feels more or less tired.

" There is no doubt that simple food is the best."

IV
PHYSICAL PERFECTION AND STRENGTH

I NOW propose to lay before you my own views as to the most direct method of gaining physical perfection, strength, and dexterity. There are a good many works in existence on training and physical culture, especially in England. Among these there are some very useful ones, but I have missed in most of them certain rules which are indispensable for the attainment of a high degree of strength. I do not propose to weary you with strange expressions and scientific language, but I wish to make you acquainted with a system to which I owe my own strength, and under which ALL other well-known strong men have trained.

In the first instance, I would have you observe the following very important rules, the neglect of which in any system, even my own, would decrease its value:—

DO YOU WISH TO BECOME STRONG?

Certainly, you will answer, that is my intention, that is my wish; to which I should reply that a simple wishing will not do it. You must want to—in other words, you must act.

You have no idea how much stress I lay on this first condition! The will I should call that incessant inward impulse which spurs one on to the goal. The beginning is difficult, and many a man gets no further than the initial stages. He is not unlike the would-be piano virtuoso, who, after a few lessons, comes to the point when the exercises become more difficult and tedious, when he throws them up altogether. Others, again, put exercises off from day to day by taking firm mental resolutions to begin in earnest and to make up for lost time, on the morrow— which seldom comes.

The question whether anyone can become strong I answer emphatically in the affirmative. I could mention dozens of cases where men of an already advanced age (40 to 60), and under the most difficult circumstances, have acquired quite a considerable increase ofstrength by physical culture.

I have already pointed out that increase of strength means betterment of health and increase of comfort, so that every man must profit by such increase of strength, even if he does not intend to acquire it for professional or other pecuniary purposes.

Believe me, excuses which a man may advance, such as, " I am too old," " I have not sufficient time," " My position or my business does not permit," etc., are all mere subterfuges to cover a weak will power. You Britons have a splendid proverb, " Where there's a will there's a way," and I am a stanch believer in it.

Now, I quite admit that to produce an extraordinarily strong man (or woman) very many favorable conditions are necessary, but I sincerely trust that the coming generation will average a physical perfection such as that now displayed by athletes, and if so this will be due to the rational physical culture and care of the body, which deservedly finds every day fresh adherents.

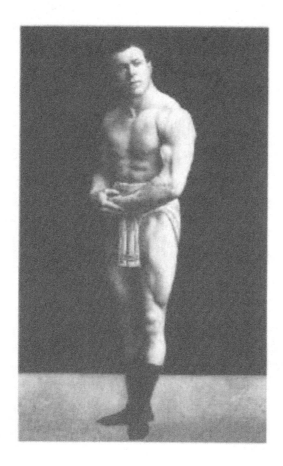

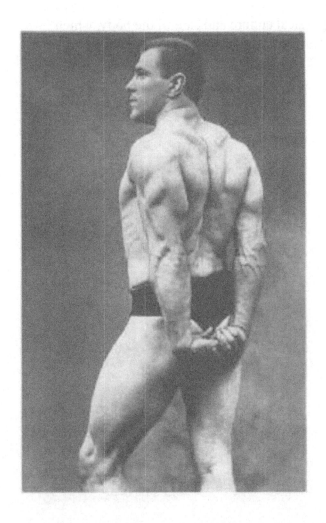

The determination to become strong is indispensable for success, and the best proof of this is that among the masses of hard toilers, however strange it may seem, we do not find very strong people, certainly not in the measure one might expect. As a wrestler, I have had an opportunity of discovering strong men in all positions of life. Manual labor alone is therefore not the source of strength. All prominent strong men have fostered their strength by the aid of a strong will power; they wanted to become strong, and consequently succeeded.

I remember a photographer in Germany who confessed to me that although in his youth he was a great enthusiast for physical culture, yet, when he realized that he would have to be a conscript, the idea of which was not only distasteful but even dreadful to him, he neglected the exercises he had once pursued, with the absolute intention of becoming, unfit and exempt from service—in which he succeeded. Here is a case of a man who wished not to be strong, and who exerted his will power to that end. The result he attained was, that from his appearance I should call him a withered individual, If a man can to such an extent exercise his will against nature, how much more can he do so to foster a natural process?

As further evidence of the influence of the " Will to Develop Weakness," may be instanced the case of the Russian Jews, among whom military service is most unpopular.

In fact the vast majority of Russian Jews seek to evade their military service, by every means in their power, and find that the only really efficacious method is by being physically unfit.

Now, as is well known, the Jews as a people are one of the healthiest in the world, and one, moreover, which has turned out a very large number of prominent athletes. The Jew, as a man, is usually quite up to the average degree of physical fitness, but the Russian Jews by the deliberate neglect of every species of physical exercise and by means of an absolute determination to become weak, manage to get themselves rejected as soldiers, in numbers out of all proportion to the relative size of their community.

" Wer will kann " (he who has the will has the power) was the motto of Herr Unthan, the man without arms, who succeeded in developing his feet in such a manner that he could use them to better advantage than many a clever man can use his hands. Another similar case is the one of Miss Rapin, the clever Swiss painter and artist, who was born without arms. My readers probably know of numerous similar cases.

Again, I have come across many young men, who by nature seemed very weak, but who, in consequence of physical exercises and a strong will power, became prominently strong.

You must have faith in your ability to make yourself strong.

It has already been proved at the present day that thought constitutes real power. A very clever apparatus has been invented, and is in existence, called the "musclebed." This automatically registers which parts of the body are provided with a more liberal flow of blood, by the simple impulse, will or thought of the person measured. Consequently, it is by no means immaterial how and what one thinks.

Banish, therefore, all your sad or miserable thoughts, and keep on with your physical training, without ever thinking for one moment that you might not succeed.

GOVERN YOUR THOUGHTS

This rule is absolutely necessary in all stages of life if you wish to succeed, for without concentration of thought, you are courting failure. How many people are there who are, so to speak, the shuttlecock of their thoughts! Every moment hundreds of ideas or thoughts rush through their brain, causing an expenditure of energy without adequate return in results. Just fancy a man at the Bisley rifle range taking aim and shooting at the same moment as he thinks of something quite different. Do you think he will carry off the King's prize, or, indeed, any prize? No, he will not even hit the target. If, therefore, you wish to become healthy and strong, you must give your thoughts to the full and without restriction in this direction, even to the most insignificant performances of your daily life. Concentrate your mind upon the idea of acquiring health and strength!

To give a few examples. The ordinary mortal may be reading his daily paper or book while taking his meals; his mind is occupied with what he is reading, instead of being bent on acquiring nourishment. He neglects proper mastication of his food, hence arise—indigestion, non- assimilation of food, bad teeth, and other ailments. Many people who suffered from painful chronic indigestion have been cured of it by the simple remedy, however strange it sounds: thorough mastication. Another man will train for years according to a fairly good method, but he neglects to devote his mind to his movements. Instead of clinging to the one important thought, " I will become strong," or " I will strengthen this particular muscle," he allows his thoughts to be distracted from the main point; the result is useless training, simply manual labor without increase of strength, but, perhaps, decrease. Every wrestler will admit that thoughts are powers; whilst one is measuring one's strength and skill with an opponent, one's thoughts must be concentrated on the game, otherwise defeat is certain. A wrestler whose attention or thought is distracted, invariably loses.

As I mentioned before, it has been proved by experiments that thought can influence a livelier rush of blood to certain parts of the body, hence the hot head and cold feet of the brain worker.

A physical culture pupil will profit by this knowledge, and avoid, for instance, erotic thoughts, for he who has erotic thoughts steers his blood into organs which are superfluous for our purpose, instead of into the arms and legs, which he intends to, and should, make strong.

One ought to avoid all unnecessary worry and exciting thoughts, and to cultivate a firm tranquility of mind. I have formed the conviction that all unnecessary sorrows and cares act in all circumstances harmfully upon one's constitution. Melancholy reflections will in no way influence Fate, whereas one may weaken the constitution by the waste of energy while indulging in them. The best is to do one's duty conscientiously, and to leave the rest to Him who guides our destiny.

He who wants to become strong can succeed in conquering his failings and mastering his shortcomings by regulating his life accordingly.

HINDRANCES TO THE ACQUISITION OF STRENGTH

Under this heading I would include the consumption of alcohols and tobacco, coffee, etc. Alcohol is, in my opinion, a nerve poison, which is not assimilated and requires a great expenditure of energy for its excretion. Furthermore, it decreases energy and deadens certain inner forces, of which we may be unconscious and which otherwise may be of great service to us. For instance, we may be tired, that is, our senses bid us leave off and rest, and thus collect fresh natural energy. But under the influence of alcohol, we are easily induced to act against our natural instinct, and as each action is followed by a reaction, the latter shows itself in various disagreeable and eventually harmful shapes, depression of spirit, bad humor, bad digestion, loss of appetite, and so forth. Alcohol therefore, or any similar stimulant which has an unnatural effect, must be injurious.

The consumption of tobacco is the most useless vice which exists. Nicotine is a direct poison to the heart, and, like alcohol, is very harmful.

I will admit that I can see no crime in an occasional indulgence in a glass of wine or a cigar; the main point is simply to be able to keep one's body and mind under full control. You may compare the connection of body and mind or soul to that between the mesmerist and his medium. It is a well-known fact that the oftener the medium submits to the will of the mesmerist the more easily the state of hypnotism is reached. If, therefore, the mind or soul submits to the suggestions of the weaker organ, the body, which bids him to have a smoke now and again, to neglect physical exercise to-day, or to indulge to excess for once in alcoholic drink, the morrow will repeat this suggestion with easier and possibly increased success. Hence to obey your body weakens the will, whilst to control it gives one strength of mind.

Moderation in sexual intercourse is very important. Sexual abstemiousness should be strictly observed during the early age of manhood and development. He who observes this recommendation will soon benefit by the immense prerogatives of chastity. A few years ago a colleague of mine said to me: " Nonsense, that is only human nature." This "clever" man, however, reached only a secondary position as a strong man, and now, at the age of thirty, he is actually degenerating as an athlete. Coffee is a stimulant and, as such, would be better avoided entirely.

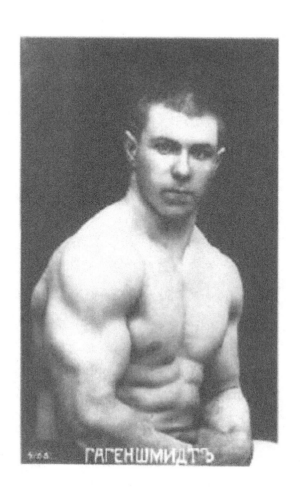

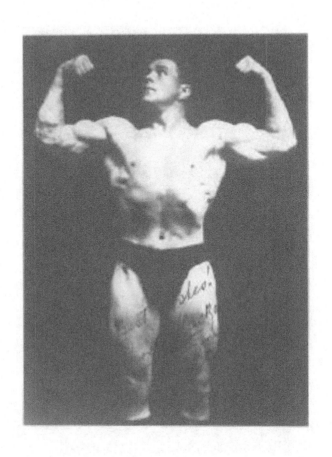

V
NUTRITION

I COME now to the much discussed subject:

WHAT OUGHT WE TO EAT?

I believe I am right in asserting that our Creator has provided food and nutriment for every being for its own advantage. Man is born without frying-pan or stewpot. The purest natural food for human beings would, therefore, be fresh, uncooked food and nuts. It is not my intention to discuss here the old problem, whether meat is necessary as food for man or whether man was created and should remain a vegetarian. My experience has taught me, that foodstuffs are of secondary importance. There are very strong people who are strict vegetarians, whilst others eat a good deal of meat. A fare which consists of three-quarters of vegetable food and one-quarter meat would appear to be the most satisfactory for the people of central Europe.

Everyone should and can find out which diet best suits his constitution, and he should avoid all food which disagrees with it. I would shun altogether all highly seasoned and sour dishes. Much has been said lately in praise of sugar as food, but as artificial sugar is an acid- forming substance, I should not recommend it. Natural sugar, such as is contained in dates, figs, and other fruit, is certainly preferable. Highly flavored or seasoned food produces thirst and therefore acts harmfully.

HOW MUCH SHOULD WE EAT?

I maintain that it is absolutely a mistake to eat a great deal. Excess is harmful, as all food which the stomach only partly digests, transforms itself in the stomach or in the intestines into poisonous matter, which in time sets up bodily decay. It is true that to a certain extent digestion improves as muscle strength increases, but even in such cases the progress may not be sufficient for a thorough assimilation of the extra food.

The disadvantages of meat foods are, in my opinion, in the first place, that nowadays it is most difficult to obtain meat from absolutely healthy animals (I count those artificially fed in stables and pens among the unhealthy ones), and, secondly, that far too much flesh food is taken.

In the case of pure vegetable food, excess is less dangerous. All food, with perhaps the exception of pure vegetables, which certainly form the ideal human food, deposits drossy sediments in the body, which may be removed by four channels, the lungs, the skin, the kidneys, and the intestines. If these four channels are in good working order, the man is healthy.

THE PRINCIPAL FOOD FOR MAN IS PURE AIR

Partake of it as much as you possibly can, breathe much, and as deeply as you can, through the nose. Breathing through the nose is the only proper way of respiration and at the same time an important regulator for the movement of the body, for, if for any kind of work the breath through the nose ceases to be sufficient, one ought to either discontinue the work or restrict the movement until breathing has again become normal.

Various deep breathing exercises are recommended by professors and other so-called authorities on Physical Culture matters.

Not wishing to be dragged into any discussion I will refrain from criticizing these, and will confine myself to strongly recommending all my readers to content themselves with the simplest and most natural deep-breathing exercise in existence. One which everyone can practise, without trouble, and which requires no argument to demonstrate its superiority over all others.

This consists simply of running exercise in the open air. Run as much as you can and as often as you can, and whenever you come across a hill, run up it. This will force you to inhale deep breaths and will also accustom you to breathe through your nose. Besides the chest and lung development resulting therefrom, you will soon appreciate the benefits which your leg muscles will derive.

I cannot lay too great stress upon the great usefulness of proper breathing, by which means we introduce into our system the essential oxygen and discharge a quantity of waste matter.

The skin of most people is in a very neglected state. In consequence of unsuitable clothing or imperfect cleansing of the countless pores, the poisonous residues cannot be expelled through the skin. These impurities consequently accumulate in the region of other outlets, such as the kidneys; if these are in good order, the function intended for the skin may be in part performed by them, but if this state of things continues, kidney disorders are sure to appear, just as skin disease will come if the kidneys and intestines work badly, and then the patient generally and foolishly tries to cure or improve the skin with salves or cosmetics.

For these reasons it must be obvious that running is a far more satisfactory breathing exercise than the mere filling and emptying of the lungs before an open window, the accompanying exertion compelling the discharge of these impurities in the form of perspiration. An important item of physical culture, indeed, is a regular care of the skin. One or two weekly baths and daily rubbing of the whole body are necessary. As to the temperature of the water, you must use your own judgment. He who dives into cold water or takes a cold douche when he is hot, or perspiring, suppresses forcibly the action of the pores and exposes himself to illness. As we are all more or less the opposite to hardy, such violent attempts at " hardening ourselves " act detrimentally on our health. Swimming is very useful, but I should not advise a longer stay in the water than one quarter of an hour at a time, as the temperature of the body becomes so low that a great amount of energy has to be expended specially to raise the warmth of the body again. When training, a cold morning bath of one half to one minute's duration before commencing will be found very beneficial. If at all possible, expose the naked body to the sun. Man is a creature of light and air, and I should therefore recommend little or no clothing when training.

WHAT WE SHOULD DRINK

In this, excess is also prejudicial, first, because one gives the kidneys more work than they were intended for, and, secondly, the very important mineral salts which the body requires for nourishment are carried away by the extra liquid. According to the discoveries of the German, Julius Hensel, it is just the presence in the body of these mineral salts, such as iron, lime, sodium, phosphorus, sulphur, chlorides and bromides, which supports energy and vital power, and if they are wanting, decay of tissue and decomposition take place. The invigorating action of sea air is partly due to the copious amount of salts and mineral matter it contains.

A German proverb says rightly:
" He who drinks and has no thirst, Or who eats and has no hunger, Unlike him whose health is first, Suffers illness and dies younger."

It is said that a large percentage of America's population suffers from weak or diseased stomachs through partaking of highly seasoned foods, or from kidney complaints through indulgence in iced drinks. It is very unwise to drink anything cold if one's body is overheated; one ought to take small mouthfuls, and swallow each only after having warmed it in one's mouth. I need not occupy space in dilating on the well-known pernicious effect of too hot liquids upon teeth and stomach.

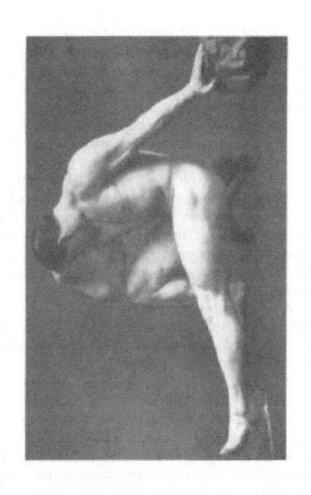

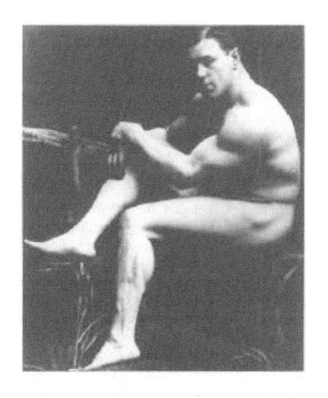

VI
REST AND WHOLESOME SLEEP

THE natural invigorating remedy for an exhausted body is rest, both in the physical as in the mental direction, and a healthy sleep. This is the only means by which the various organs and muscles may rid themselves of the " fatigue poison " and collect and develop fresh energy.

I have already touched on the necessity of controlling one's thoughts and the method of doing so, and would now refer to a few dispositions of mind which are very detrimental; these are excitement, worry, fretting and anger. Avoid violent emotion, also gambling, worry about unavoidable or unalterable situations, etc. All these emotions draw blood into the brain, and thus cause a weakening of the other organs used for work and movement. Be careful in the choice of literature. Here also avoid excess and especially erotic novels.

To obtain a sound sleep, the regulation of the proper functions of the intestines and the skin is necessary above everything else.

He who takes daily and thorough exercise in the open will hardly be plagued by sleeplessness. It is advisable to observe as far as possible regular hours for sleep. Sleep during night is better than during daytime. Seven to nine hours suffice amply, and here again too much is unwholesome. Nervous people, or those who work much with the brain, would do well to rest once or twice a day for about one quarter to half an hour after a meal.

DWELLING ROOMS

Unhealthy dwelling rooms are very injurious. Bedrooms, in particular, should be well-ventilated and exposed to sunlight. I should recommend every father of a family to arrange his dwelling so that the largest and best situated rooms are used as bedrooms, seeing that one-third of one's life is spent there.

Damp walls, damp bed clothes, and the like are to be rigorously avoided, and care in this direction cannot be too greatly insisted upon. The least evils which they bring are gout, rheumatism, colds, etc.

Heavy curtains in bedrooms should be avoided, also large carpets, which cannot easily be cleaned. Both harbor dust and impurities. Small curtains should frequently be washed.

CLOTHING

Clothes should not be too warm nor too tight, in order to allow free action to the function of the skin, and to the development of the several parts of the body. Corsets and tight boots are no good for a physical culturist. A very good material for clothing, if it were not too dear, is silk; after this comes good linen (most suitable for underwear), wool, and cotton.

I have now made mention of the principal items which act beneficially or detrimentally upon the physical development of man, among which there are many recommendations with which the reader is no doubt familiar, but which cannot be repeated too often. I admit that these counsels may seem superfluous to some, but their careful observance will help one to not only keep well, but to gain the physical strength which, I believe, to be the goal of my readers.

I have come across all sorts and conditions of people among the many who have asked my advice or opinion on different subjects, and on my own principles for the attainment of the strength and muscular development which gained for me such reputation as I may possess, either as a wrestler or as an athlete.

I have seen would-be athletes, who cared most for the exterior of their bodies, and others who were faddists or cranks; these people would try all sorts of novelties in dress, diet, apparatus, food, etc. They fell from one extreme into the other, and believed that they could become strong by easy and comfortable means, forgetting that there are only two principal means of acquiring strength—exercise and perseverance.

VII
TRAINING

BEFORE I describe what I consider the best method of training for the acquisition of strength, I should like to make a few remarks with regard to its application.

It stands to reason that the natural bent and abilities for physical development in different people vary with the individual. An old man will have to train differently from a young man, a woman differently from a child, while there are various gradations for age and sex. There are, however, a great many people who seem to be hindered by their vocation or calling from a methodical training on these lines. To these I would say that there is always some time available every day which can be devoted to physical exercises and the care of the body. If you wish to become strong and well, you must attend to this, just as you must find time for eating. And, again, if you do not find time to become and remain healthy, you will be obliged to find time to be ill. Surely some of the hours wasted on banal and often harmful pleasures might be devoted to physical exercise.

Of course, I am aware that there are people whose occupation is very trying, and others who undergo great mental strain. I should recommend such to study and follow particularly the part of my book dealing with the mastery and concentration of thought while they are training, when their success will be certain. Brain workers must, however, proceed with particular care, following the maxim, " Slowly but surely." They will require months where others require weeks owing to their more favorable conditions; but the result will be the same.

THE BEST METHOD OF TRAINING

As a principal rule I should stipulate for regularity of training. Any observant student will have noticed that the mechanism of the body reacts unconsciously, and with an often surprising punctuality, consequent upon certain repeated activity, by reason of its habit and adaptability. For instance, if one follows a regular mode of life, one wakens always at the same hour; hunger and vigor, etc., are also similarly experienced at certain times of the day. Hence it is advisable to exercise as nearly as possible at the same hour every day. The time will, of course, vary with different people. I should not advise the practice of physical exercise, more particularly exercise with weights, in the morning immediately after rising, as most people are not then particularly vigorous. The best time is during the two hours previous or subsequent to a principal meal; if before, one ought to leave off at least a quarter of an hour before eating, so that the nerves may become calm, otherwise loss of appetite may be entailed.

The exercises should not exceed one quarter of an hour at the commencement, and should only be increased by five minutes in a few months. Afterwards, about thirty minutes are fully sufficient to the acquisition and preservation of strength and endurance.

Another useful point to notice is that it is unadvisable to sit down and rest between the exercises, as not only is one likely to contract a chill by so doing, but the muscles themselves will become stiff and contracted.

You will naturally be wearing a minimum of clothing while exercising, so as soon as you have run through one series, throw a towel or wrap over your shoulders and walk briskly up and down the room. This will keep the blood circulating and rebuilding the consumed tissue. It will also assist the process of perspiration or discharge of waste matter and will above all assist in the maintenance of looseness and suppleness in joint, muscle and sinew so highly to be desired by the athlete whose ambition is directed towards the acquisition of health and strength and not merely that development which is intended to display itself solely before a looking-glass or camera.

All exercises should be made slowly, and with full concentration of the mind; observe by all means regular breathing, carefully waiting after every exercise until a calm respiration through the nose has again taken place.

There are certain advantages in going through the exercises with one or two companions, but if these are mere spectators, it is better to exercise alone, for fear of having one's thoughts diverted from the work.

VARIATIONS IN THE EXERCISES

It is advisable to vary the exercises constantly, so as to avoid too great a strain on single muscle groups, and rather to develop all muscles harmoniously.

I should like to point here to a great mistake which a vast number of thoughtless people make during training. Every human being has a certain part of his body more developed by nature than other parts; say, for instance, that the legs of one or the arms of another are naturally strong. Now, the former will be able to perform the leg exercises with perfect ease and comfort, whereas all his arm exercises require more exertion. It would be foolish if this particular individual were to devote more time and attention to his leg exercises because they are easier to him, and neglect his arm exercises, which to him are harder and more difficult. Nevertheless, this is a bad habit into which many people fall during training. While in this case the legs become stronger, the arms do not develop in the same ratio. It is, therefore, most necessary to train systematically.

Further on I shall give particulars of the various exercises, and I recommend my readers to map out a certain plan, according to which they exercise all the muscle groups twice on three or four days every week, or on six days, if time allows.

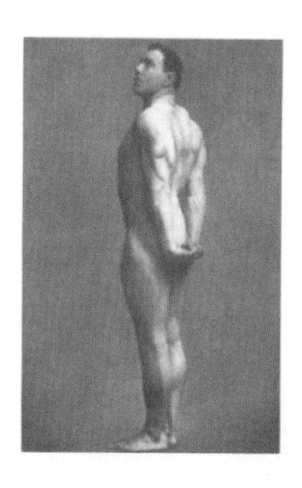

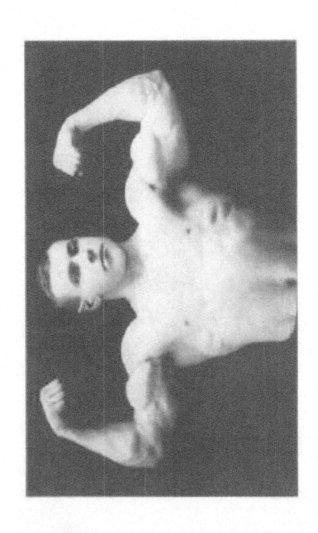

VIII
EXERCISES WITHOUT WEIGHTS

I CAN hear a few of my readers exclaiming, "These instructions are all, no doubt, excellent, but then I am not going to exercise with weights. My doctor doesn't approve of them for one thing and I myself am not particularly keen on them for another. Besides which, I travel about a good deal, attending to my business, and it would be highly inconvenient for me to have to add bar-bells, dumb-bells, etc., to my ordinary luggage."

In response to these objections, I can only say that the last one raised, does certainly possess a certain amount of force, although by purchasing a series of disc weights, the encumbrance would be reduced to a minimum in the matters of weight, bulk, and cost.

As to the others, well, it is my opinion that every one —man, woman, and child without exception—will find exercise with a graduated and suitably adapted series of weights of the utmost benefit. Nevertheless, I do not expect everyo ne to be converted to my views, however convinced I may personally be of their merit. As to medical views on the matter, well, I have had the pleasure of hearing the opinions of every leading medical authority in the world, who has really studied the matter, and they are, one and all, in agreement with those which I myself entertain and have set forth in these pages.

Medical men who are opposed to exercises with weights have never investigated them, and are totally ignorant of their value. No living person is so weak as to be unable to exercise in this fashion, all that is necessary being to graduate the weights. Even a weak heart can be strengthened by exercises with weights.

Still, I am aware there are certain people who may entertain a sentimental objection to strength, and who object, in consequence, to run any risk of acquiring a powerful muscular development. All these people are, however, anxious to preserve their own health and to avoid any necessity of incurring expense in the shape of medical attendance and drugs. As already pointed out, health cannot be divorced from strength. The body, in order to be healthy, must be strong, so that it will be found that the series of exercises, set forth in this chapter, while being free from all inconvenient possibilities of great strength development, will yet, if conscientiously practised, develop a fair average physique, as well as a sound, all-round physical fitness—in other words, a sound and healthy constitution.

There is one other reason for this chapter, or rather for the exercises detailed therein, being deserving of especial attention, and that is that these Exercises without weights should be regarded as being a preliminary course even for those ambitious of athletic renown.

Even where a youth is so naturally strong and fit that he might safely enter straight away on a course of weight- lifting exercises, and of exercises with weights, he will be well advised if he devotes at least two or three weeks to these exercises without weights, and further to include a fair selection of them in his programme of daily exercise with weights. I have myself repeated a few in my next chapter, partly as an indication of the method I would like my readers to follow, and while the ones I have repeated must on no account be neglected, I would not wish anyone to think that on this account the others may be passed over altogether.

The exercises themselves will be found to include movements which will strengthen every necessary part of the human frame, and should therefore be patronized in ratio to the actual need for same; i.e., a reader suffering or liable to attacks of indigestion, constipation or other intestinal disorders, should pay particular attention to Exercises 6, 8, 9, 10, and 13; while a reader in need of chest, neck and throat development would, on the other hand, rely mainly on Exercises 1, 2, 3,4, 5, and 14. Sufficient indications, however, are given with the exercises themselves to enable anyone to make his or her own selection.

I would, however, strongly advise one and all to pay full attention to the advice already given on the subjects of Nutrition, Rest, Breathing Exercises, etc., and to adhere as closely as possible to the lines previously laid down with regard to these points. I would also like to see a fair amount of attention paid to the exercises dealt with in Chapter IX. They may not care to carry these out with the weights recommended therewith perhaps, but there are some, notably those for neck development, chest development, strengthening the abdominal muscles, etc., which should on no account be neglected.

The weights utilized for these could be, if necessary, considerably reduced, say to a half, or even less, of the minimum advised. This will, and indeed should, depend almost entirely on the physical powers of the reader himself. I cannot pretend to be acquainted with those of each and every one. In order to institute a scale, it is only necessary to remember that the weights prescribed (save in the section for athletes) are well within the normal healthy and active man's powers, and that ladies and children, elderly and invalid readers must, to a large extent, fix the amount most suitable to themselves by an estimate formed on that basis; and, further, in making such decision, that it will be safer to underestimate rather than overestimate their own strength to commence with.

I would suggest that at least fifteen minutes be daily devoted to the system of exercises adopted, the best period being immediately after rising, subsequent to the matutinal bath.

As an alternative to the above, nightly exercise, i.e., just before retiring, is almost as good, and in certain cases (when one does not sleep well, for instance) even preferable.

Never on any account continue the exercises until exhaustion sets in and always relax your muscles afterwards, in the manner recommended in the last chapter. Further, do not devote your whole attention solely to the easiest movements. These will very probably be calculated to develop those parts in which you are already strong, whereas your chief aim should be to so strengthen your less well developed muscles, that your body may be in perfect harmony and tune.

Look upon this condition as being the goal of your ambitions, concentrate your thoughts thereon and on the muscles which your exercise is developing, thereby assisting your progress, and

TO INVALIDS AND LEISURED PERSONS

I would specially offer the recommendation that they devote several quarters of an hour daily to the practice of the majority of the exercises dealt with in this chapter.

By so doing they will (if ill) be hastening their recovery and fortifying their systems against future attacks of illness, and, all such will, in any case, be profitably employing hours which might otherwise hang somewhat heavily on their hands.

MIDDLE-AGED AND ELDERLY PEOPLE

are far too apt to imagine that for them the age of physical exercise is past. Herein they are really seriously at fault, for they are often the very people who stand most in need of such. They, for instance, are the ones most liable to suffer from superfluous adipose tissue, defective digestion and irregular circulation. They would indeed benefit considerably by the exercises detailed in Chapter IX, but as (supposing them to be commencing exercise for the first time) they will possibly shrink from the use of dumb-bells and bar-bells, I have perhaps borne them more in mind, while arranging the following series. As far as possible, therefore, should they devote their attention to these, and as soon as their interest has been sufficiently awakened enter upon the advanced course, under, of course, lighter conditions than those recommended for younger readers, with the less strenuous movements, persevering with these until they are able to practically run through the whole series.

FOURTEEN SIMPLE EXERCISES WITHOUT APPARATUS

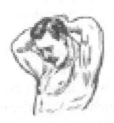 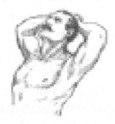

Exercise No. 1

No. 1.—Stand erect with hands clasped behind your neck. Now press the head forcibly down until the chin touches the chest, exerting the full strength of your neck muscles to resist the pressure. When the chin is down force the head back by exertion of the neck muscles against the hand pressure. Repeat this alternate movement, at first for five repetitions, gradually increasing same. Neck muscles specially.

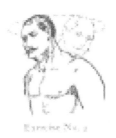
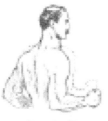

No. 2.—Stand erect and roll the head round and round by bending the neck in a circular motion. Continue for, say, ten repetitions, gradually increasing the number up to twenty. Neck muscles specially.

No. 3.—Stand erect with elbows at sides, arms bent at right angles, hands clenched. Now roll your shoulders right round if possible, back, up, forward and down. Continue until tired. Shoulder muscles specially.

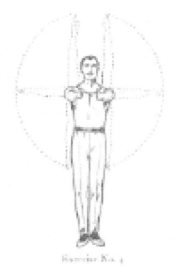

No. 4.—Stand erect, with arms stretched straight out in front of you, palms turned inwards. Force arms straight back into line with the shoulders. Raise them sideways to full stretch above head, palms to the front, and bring them down in front of you at full stretch, till the palms rest on the

front of the thighs. Return to full stretch above head and then to first position. Continue exercise for say a full minute. Chest expansion mainly.

No. 5.—Stand with right leg crossed over left, both arms crossed across chest, hands clasping shoulders. Spring out to a full stride of each leg sideways, throwing arms back, hands open, to a line with the shoulders. Return sharply and continue for twenty repetitions. All leg muscles, as well as the arms, shoulders, back and chest will be greatly benefited.

No. 6.—Stand erect with feet close together, arms and hands fully stretched above the head. Now swing the trunk right round in a circular motion (as near as possible), bending over to the right, forward, round to the left and back, waist circling or swinging from the hips only. Continue for from five to ten full circles at first, according to the ease with which the movement can be executed and increase gradually. Persevere until tired, but not as far as exhaustion. Keep arms loose. This exercise will be found specially helpful in cases of intestinal disorder, particularly when accompanied by a too extensive waist. The spine will also be considerably strengthened.

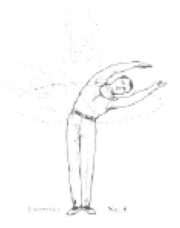

No. 7.—Stand erect, feet together, arms fully stretched, palms of hands pressed together. Then keeping all muscles taut, bend down gradually, elevating the left leg into such a position as would enable a straight line to be drawn along the back of the hands to the extended heel. Endeavour to approach as closely to this position as it is possible to assume—the knee of the supporting leg may be slightly bent if necessary in order to get as near to the desired result as possible. Go slowly back and repeat forward bend, extending right leg. Continue for five repetitions, increasing one per week to twenty repetitions. This will be found a fairly strenuous exercise, highly developing all the leg muscles. The arms, hip, back and shoulders will also derive great benefit, particularly in the extensor muscles, and if persevered with at a comparatively early age. Its influence on height may readily be observed. Besides all which the practice in the

balance and equipoise of the body cannot be overestimated.

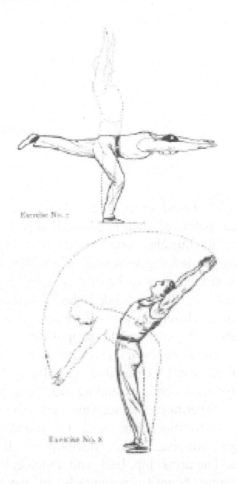

No. 8.—Stand erect, with feet slightly apart, arms fully stretched, palms facing each other. Bend right forward from the hips, as far down as possible without bending the knees, and then swing right back, as far as possible. Repeat five times each

movement alternately, increasing gradually to twenty repetitions. Abdominal and back muscles.

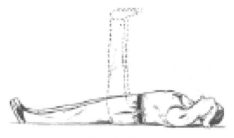

No. 9.—Lie down full length on floor as shown in sketch and raise the legs to right angles with the body. Repeat five times and increase gradually, say by one repetition a week. Abdominal, back, and hip muscles.

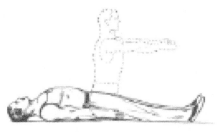

No. 10.—Lie down full length as shown and rise into sitting posture without moving the legs. This may at first necessitate a counterpoise of some sort,

such as hooking the feet under a chest of drawers or something of the kind, but persevere until you can rise without any such assistance. Repeat five times and increase gradually as last. Similar muscles affected, but in slightly different manner and proportion.

No. 11.—Stand erect, with legs crossed as shown in dotted diagram, the hands resting lightly on hips. Sweep front leg well round and to the rear, sinking the body into position of that assumed by a lady in the old-style deep courtesy. Return slowly, change legs and repeat up to five times, increasing once per week to twenty-five repetitions. Endeavour throughout to imitate closely the graceful action of the old minuet. This will be found an extremely trying exercise, especially on the leg muscles, although the abdominals will also benefit considerably.

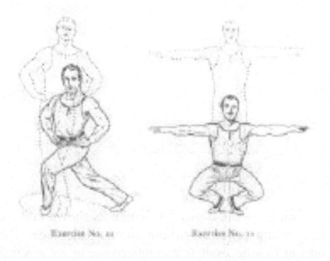

No. 12.—Stand erect, heels together, feet turned out. Extend arms right and left from shoulders and sink down, bending the knees outwards and rising on the toes, until you are almost squatting on your heels. Return to first position and repeat bend with arms stretched out in front. Return and again sink with arms stretched above head. Repeat these three performances daily for first week and then perform two of each and so on. One of the best leg exercises in the world.

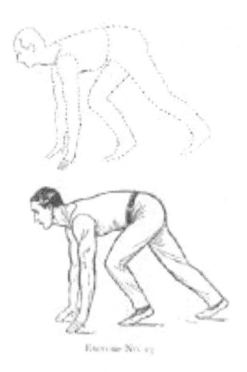

No.13.—Take up position as shown in diagram, the arms to be straight, resting on thumbs

and fingers, front leg fairly bent, back leg slightly. The weight to be chiefly supported by the arms. Then pushing off smartly with rear foot, raising the body thereby, rapidly alternate position of feet. Spring smartly each time, but not too sharply, as by doing the latter you might strain the muscles at the back of the thigh and calf. For the same reason, this exercise should not be too frequently practised; say three times per week, or rather, on alternate days. The muscles chiefly affected are both the extensors and flexors (the stretching and contracting muscles) of the thighs and calves, the abdominals, the chest, back of the neck, back and arm muscles. It is a very strengthening exercise, but at the same time somewhat exhausting, and should therefore not be repeated more than fifteen times at the first trial, thereafter to be extended to at most thirty or forty repetitions, increasing five per week.

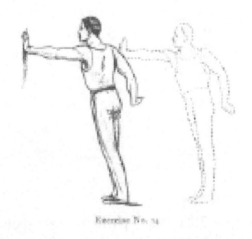

No. 14.—The following exercise, which is very popular with Turkish athletes, will be found of the utmost benefit to the arm muscles, the chest and indeed to the whole system generally. To obtain the fullest advantages, the movements should be carried out as smartly as possible. Stand about four feet from a wall (the exact distance being governed by one's height and length of reach, but in any case one should be slightly overbalanced). Lean against the wall with the full weight supported by the right hand, which is pressed against the wall, the body being slightl y turned to the left. Push off smartly so that the body sways back and turns to the right, falling towards the wall and being stayed therefrom by the rigid left arm. Push off again smartly with left and meet wall with right. Continue the exercise, as quickly as possible, until tired, gradually increasing the number of repetitions, as capacity to withstand the strain, is developed.

IX
MUSCLE EXERCISES WITH WEIGHTS

ANY male reader who is normally of good physique, who has indulged in any form of athletics, or who has practised the series of exercises dealt with in the last chapter, for a period, say, of six months, should, however, devote his principal attention to muscular development. He may secure and maintain a condition of fair physical fitness by means of exercise without weights, such exercises as have been detailed in Chapter VIII; but he cannot hope to become really strong unless he exercises with weights; for it is only by so doing that he can develop muscle of really good quality, and, as already hinted, it is important, both from the Health and the Strength points of view, that every muscular group throughout the body should be of the best quality attainable.

Every human being possesses about five hundred separate muscles, but it would be neither necessary nor useful to detail all these here.

For the purposes of development, of culture that is to say, it will be quite sufficient to classify them in groups, such as Neck muscles, Shoulder muscles, Arm muscles, Chest muscles. Muscles of the Abdomen, Back, Legs, etc.

No one can afford to neglect any of these groups. All, in fact, should be equally developed, those which are naturally weaker to greater extent than the others, until all are equally strong, when the object in view, should be that of equal all-round improvement.

To commence with the

FIRST SERIES FOR THE NECK MUSCLES

Exercise 1.—Repeat Exercise No. 1 in last chapter, i.e., place clasped hands on the back of the neck and press head downwards on chest, resisting this pressure by the exercise of the neck muscles. Commence with five repetitions, and increase gradually, say once with every third performance, up to finally twenty repetitions.

Exercise 2.—Reverse the above exercise by pressing head back against hand resistance and perform as before.

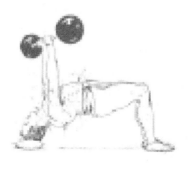

Exercise 3.—Exercise No. 2, dealt with in last chapter. Stand erect and roll head in every direction by bending the neck as much as possible. Continue as directed in Exercise 1.

Exercise 4.—Press a bar-bell weighing from 30 lb. to 50 lb. with both hands into the head bridge, as shown in sketch.

Place a rather hard cushion under the head (a rolled-up coat or the like, if nothing else is available). The body should rest on the heels and crown of the head only.

At first this exercise may not be found easy of accomplishment, in which case the bridge should be perfected before the bar-bell press is attempted. The higher the bridge, the easier will the press be found.

Repeat three times to commence with and gradually increase, say once every second week, up to ten repetitions ; then add 5 lb. to bell and commence again with three repetitions and so on.

A capital exercise for strengthening the muscles of the neck, nape and spine.

Exercise 5.—Get down on hands and knees and hang, by a broad belt, a weight on the back of the head (at first 10 lb. would be sufficient). With this move the head up, down and to both sides until tired, but not exhausted.

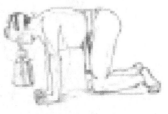

SECOND SERIES FOE THE NECK, SHOULDER, ARM, AND CHEST MUSCLES

IN most systems of Physical Culture I have observed the shoulder muscles seem sadly neglected, and that therefore many otherwise well-developed athletes have narrow and unshapely shoulders. I would therefore wish to see special attention devoted to those exercises in this section, which deal principally with the shoulders.

It will have been observed that Exercises 4 and 5 just dealt with exert a beneficial influence on the shoulder muscles (as will many others), but this must on no account be considered as sufficient, and it is because the first three of the present series directly affect the shoulders that I would like to see them regularly practised.

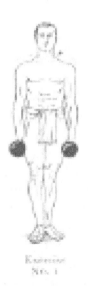

Exercise 1.—Stand erect as in sketch, holding a 10 lb. dumb-bell in each hand. Hunch shoulders as high as possible for ten repetitions, increasing by one with every third performance of exercise up to twenty repetitions; then increase weights by 5 lb. and commence afresh.

Exercise 2.—Then holding arms bent at elbows roll the shoulders right round and repeat as in last exercise.

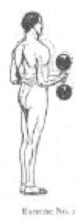 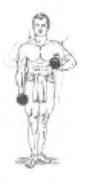

Exercise 3.—Standing erect with 5 lb. dumb-bell in each hand, hanging at sides, raise same smartly to armpits, each hand alternately, as shown in sketch. Commence with five repetitions, adding one every week up to ten. Then add 1 lb. to each dumb-bell and commence afresh, and so on.

Exercise 4.—Jerk with both arms from the shoulders a bar-bell of from 30 lb. to 50 lb. in weight, using arm strength only. Jerk both with top and bottom holds, five times each to commence with, adding one repetition per week up to ten. Then add 10 lb. to the bell and commence afresh.

Top hold means with the back of the hand pointing upward, as against bottom hold when the back of the hand points downwards.

NOTE.—For all these exercises where an approximate weight is given the following chapter on " Weights for Exercises " should be consulted.

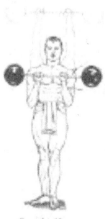

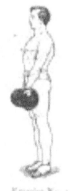

Exercise 5.—Pull up with both hands, top hold, a barbell of from 10 lb. to 15 lb., from the hang to the shoulders as shown in sketch. The elbows should be held firmly against the sides, the lift to be performed without any movement of the body. Repeat five times, increasing by one every week up to ten times. Then add 5 lb. and commence afresh.

(ii) This exercise should also be performed with bottom hold, beginning with from 20 lb. to 25 lb., for five repetitions and continuing as with top hold.

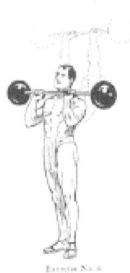

Exercise 6.—Press a bar-bell of from 30 lb. to 50 lb. from shoulders to full arm's length above the head. Begin with five repetitions, increasing by one every week up to ten. Then add 5 lb. to weight and commence afresh. This exercise is to be performed with both top and bottom holds.

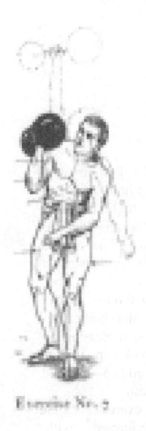

Exercise No. 7

Exercise 7.—Jerk a bar-bell of from 25 lb. to 40 lb. from the shoulder, erect above the head, with one arm.

The elbow should rest firmly against the hip, thus transferring the whole weight of the bar-bell to the legs, principally to the one leg. Quickly bend the knees, and, at the same time, " throw " the weight upwards, while with the same quick movement you stretch the arm. You will find that the principal impetus of strength will be given by the legs. The movements have to be made very quickly.

This particular exercise requires a certain technique. It greatly furthers the preservation of a perfect nimbleness and equilibrium, and develops at the same time the muscles of the legs, forearm, and triceps.

The exercise should be performed with both the right and the left arm, at first five times, every second week increasing by one up to ten times, then increase weight by 5 lb. and start afresh.

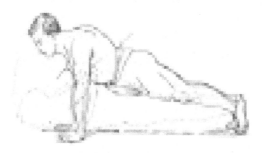

Exercise 8.—Parallel bar exercise between two chairs without weight.

This exercise can also be performed on the floor, but the body must be kept perfectly rigid. Thus, forearm, shoulder, and abdominal muscles are brought into play. Begin with five repetitions, and increase by one every week, up to twenty repetitions.

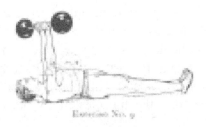

Exercise 9.—Lying on the floor, press with both arms with top hold a bar-bell of from 30 lb. to 50 lb. for five repetitions when exercising. Increase by one every week up to ten times, then add 10 lb. and start afresh. This exercise should also be done with bottom hold.

Exercise 10.—Swing a bar-bell of from 15 lb. to 30 lb., with straight arms and top hold, from the thigh to full arms' length above the head. Repeat five times, increasing by one every week up to ten repetitions, then increase weight by 5 lb. and start afresh.

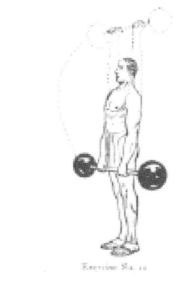

Exercise No. 11

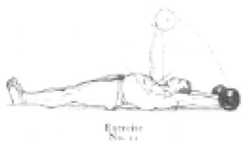

Exercise No. 11

Exercise 11.—Lying down full length on the floor, pull over the head with stretched arms to a line with the shoulders a bar-bell of from 10 lb. to 20 lb. Repeat five times, increasing by one repetition every week up to ten repetitions, and then increase weight by 5 lb. and start afresh.

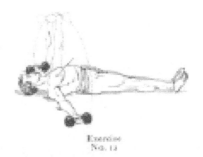

Exercise 12.—Lying down as before, with arms outstretched sideways, lift to arm's length in front of body a 10 lb. dumb-bell in each hand. Repeat five times, increasing by one repetition every week up to ten times, then increase weight of dumb-bells 1 lb. each and start afresh.

THIRD SERIES OF EXERCISES FOR DEVELOPING THE ABDOMINAL, BACK AND HIP MUSCLES PRINCIPALLY

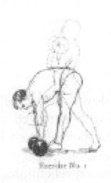
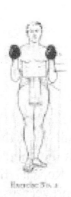

Exercise 1.—Stoop down and pull in to the chest a bar-bell of, say, 30 lb. with top hold. Straighten the shoulders well during the movement. Repeat five times, increasing by one every week up to ten repetitions and then add 5 lb. and start afresh.

Exercise 2.—Stoop down as before and pull in with each hand a 20 lb. dumb-bell, simultaneously. Repeat five times, increasing as before to ten times, then add 5 lb. to each bell and start afresh.

Exercise 3.—Press a bar-bell of from 10 lb. to 20 lb. full reach above the head; then bend forward as shown in sketch. Repeat five times at first, increasing by one every week up to ten repetitions. Then increase weight by 5 lb. and start afresh.

The hip, abdominal and back muscles are all well benefited by this exercise.

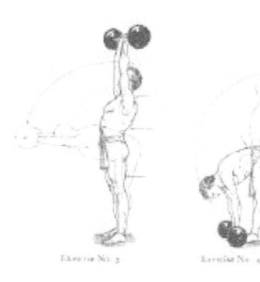

Exercise 4.—Stoop down and pull up to " hang," as shown in sketch, a bar-bell of from 50 lb. to 70 lb. with both hands (top hold), arms and legs to be perfectly straight. See that the hip muscles alone are exercised. Commence with five repetitions, increasing gradually say by one per week up to ten; then increase weight by 10 lb. and start afresh.

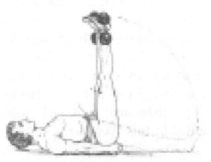

Exercise 5.—Lie down full length on your back and raise both legs, forming a right angle with the body. Repeat five times, adding one repetition weekly up to ten repetitions. Then commence afresh, tying 5 lb. to each foot.

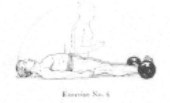

Exercise 6.—Lie down full length as in last exercise and rise into sitting posture without moving the legs. At first it may be necessary to establish a counterpoise by laying a bar-bell over the feet or legs. Repeat five times, increasing as in last up to ten. Then hold a 5 lb. weight against forehead and commence afresh. This weight can afterwards be increased gradually by holding a dumbbell in each hand close to the head.

A GRIP EXERCISE FOR DEVELOPING THE STRENGTH OF THE HANDS, FOREARMS, ETC.

FOR HOME USE Get a round stick, a thick broom-handle will do, although it should be from 1 in. to 1½ in. thick. Pierce a hole through this and suspend by a cord a 5 lb. weight. Now stand on two chairs and, holding the bar waist high, roll it round with both hands, winding up the cord. Continue until the weight is wound close up and then unwind to full length. Both wind and unwind with continuous and also with reverse rollings. Continue until tired. The rolling movement to be always steady and gradual.

FOR GYMNASIUM USE For use in gymnasia, schools, etc., a special stand may be constructed, as shown in sketch. In this instance, two weights should be used attached to each end of the bar. Five pounds' weight each will be found more than ample to commence with. The rollings to be performed as for Home use, but the bar is, of course, now supported.

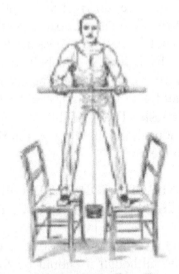

Grip Exercise for Home Use

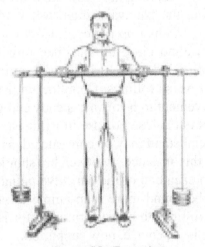

Arranged for Gymnasium

FOURTH SERIES OF EXERCISES FOR SPECIALLY DEVELOPING THE LEG MUSCLES

A note of warning should here be sounded, to the effect that, while everyone suffering from rupture, or with a tendency to rupture, should be very careful in all exercises, they must be particularly so with leg exercises. These would do well, in fact, to confine their leg movements to those without weights, and in any event to avoid altogether Exercise 5 set forth below.

Nevertheless, if the reader be sound and fit and free from such local weakness as might possibly terminate in rupture, then should he on no account neglect any of the leg exercises; for it must be remembered that while walking, cycling, etc., are good exercises for the leg muscles, yet are they insufficient alone to develop them satisfactorily for the performance of either weight-lifting feats or even of heavy weight-lifting exercises.

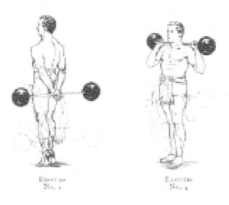

Exercise 1.—Hold a bar-bell of from 10 lb. to 20 lb. weight behind the back with arms crossed, heels together, toes pointed outwards. Now make a deep knee bend, rising on your toes, parting your knees, until almost squatting on your heels. Rise again to first position. Repeat five times, adding one repetition per week up to twenty repetitions, after which increase weight by 5 lb. and start afresh. (This exercise is called " Hacke " in Germany).

Exercise 2.—Jumping. Take running and standing high and long jumps, but standing jumps particularly. Jump with and without weights and also practise hop, step and jump; three forward jumps; hop, cross and jump, and all the Lancashire varieties.

Exercise 3.—Skipping exercise, especially with long runs on the toes of one foot, which will be found particularly beneficial to the calf muscles.

Exercise 4.—Hold a bar-bell of from 20 lb. to 40 lb. weight with both hands on the shoulders, behind the neck, feet together, and make the deep knee bend without raising the heels. This exercise will specially develop the muscles of the thighs and groin. Commence with three repetitions, increasing by one every week up to ten repetitions, after which add 5 lb. and commence afresh.

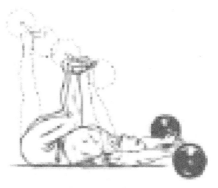

Exercise No. 5

Exercise 5.—Lying full length on the floor on your back, raise your legs well over to an acute angle with your body, bending both at your hips and knees. Pull over your head a bar-bell of from 20 lb. to 30 lb. and rest it across the soles of your feet. When this has been well balanced, push your legs straight, bend them in again, and again push straight. Repeat at first from three to five times according to ability, gradually increasing until ten repetitions can be made fairly easily, when add 5 lb. weight and start afresh.

(N.B.—The weight used and number of repetitions recommended for this exercise can only be approximate. The first essential is to secure and maintain a perfect balance, wherefor a very light bar-bell indeed may beused until a perfect equilibrium has been secured.)

X
WEIGHTS FOR EXERCISES

WHAT WEIGHT SHOULD ONE EXERCISE WITH?

SOME trainers recommend to their pupils for the training of all muscle groups one and the same (light) weight and believe they are able to obtain the same effect by frequent repetitions.

My experience has taught me that this is wrong, for the muscles of men or animals who are distinguished for certain feats of endurance are by no means over-developed. A long-distance runner or long-distance cyclist always has comparatively thin legs, as have a racehorse, stag, or greyhound. Nature does not act without aim and purpose. Hence there is a great difference between feats of endurance and feats of strength. One must consider that, although it is quite possible to enlarge muscles by certain light, prolonged exercises, at the same time the development of the sinews may be neglected, and it is the sinews which transport the action of the muscles to the bone frame. The sinews can only be exercised and strengthened by correspondingly heavy muscle work. Besides, to take a paradoxical example, it is quite impossible to improve strong muscle groups, as, for instance, the hip muscles, with light-weight exercises.

A further illustration of the fallacy of attempting to develop the muscles by frequent repetitions with the same light exercises may be found in a comparison with any and every other form of athletics, in which a man would never think of merely repeating his training programme. In order to improve himself either in pace or distance, he must set himself a steady progression of arduous effort.

HOW CAN ONE GAUGE THE MOST SUITABLE WEIGHTS FOR EXERCISE?

This is quite easy. When in an unfatigued condition try an exercise say ten times. If you can accomplish this by using all your strength you have found the proper weight with which to begin your exercises five times in succession.

HOW TO INCREASE THE WEIGHTS AND THE NUMBER OF MOVEMENTS

After having ascertained the correct weight for every exercise, begin each movement, say five times, and increase the number by one every week: thus five one week, six the next, seven the next, etc., until the prescribed maximum is reached. After that begin afresh with a weight that is 5 lb. heavier for one arm exercises, or 10 lb. for two arms, unless otherwise directed.

WHEN SHOULD ONE BEGIN TRIALS WITH HEAVY WEIGHTS?

This should only be done after one has trained for at least three months in the foregoing manner with light weights, and one should never begin to lift any heavier weight than one can lift without much exertion at least ten times.

He who ventures such trials without this previous training exposes himself to strainings or breakings of the sinews or muscles, also to ruptures, and I would particularly caution my readers against any such imprudent experiments.

I strongly recommend at the beginning of training the recording in a book, say every three months, of one's measurements and weights, also of the progress made. The measurements which should be taken are of the following parts: neck (thinnest part); forearm (thinnest part); forearm (thickest part), the arm to be held out and only the fist closed; biceps of arm held straight out; biceps of arm bent; the forearm and biceps measurements to be taken right and left; chest (normal, measured across the nipples); chest (deflated); chest (inflated); wrist (normal); thigh (thickest part); leg (just above the knee); calf.

Always take the measurements before any exercises.

It is a fact that the first improvement which the muscles undergo is in their quality long before they grow in size. It therefore follows that if the muscles are of fatty or watery nature a diminution in the size of some of them will take place. This is quite a natural consequence, which must be borne in mind, and which must not discourage the pupil in the least

After exercising when undressed, one ought to try by the straining of certain muscle groups to obtain a fine molding of one's body and a complete mastery over single parts of it. In other words, you must practise posing for effect.

XI
EXERCISES FOR ATHLETES

AFTER having trained three or four months, on the system dealt with in the last chapter, a great increase of strength will be soon perceived. If it is intended to further increase it, one should begin to train once or twice per week (provided always one does not possess any tendency to rupture) with heavier weights. I recommend the use for six months only of such weights as one can handle at least five to ten times for one exercise, and on such days avoid part, if not all, ordinary exercises.

There are a great many weight-lifting exercises, which might be mentioned, but I propose here to confine myself to the principal ones for ordinary feats of strength. The bar-bell for this purpose should be 1 in. thick.

Always take a deep breath before each separate lift. Do not wear a tight belt when practising.

1. SNATCH WITH ONE HAND (right or left).

Rule: The bar-bell is lifted with one hand without stop from floor to full extent above the head.

Execution: Place the bar-bell near both feet over the instep, get hold precisely in the middle, bend down, lay the free hand on the respective knee (left hand on the left knee or right hand on the right knee), take a quick and firm grip, and pull the weight at the same time with a lightning rapidity upwards. The muscles of the hand, forearms, biceps, shoulders, legs, abdomen, and hip should all work together only for a fraction of a second (perhaps hardly one-tenth of a second) to obtain a good result.

Many athletes snatch the bar only up to the eyes, after which they get their body underneath like lightning. This indicates great strength of legs and agility.

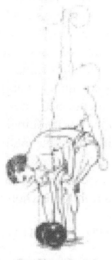

One Hand Snatch

Several French and German athletes snatch about 180 lb. with one hand. Formerly, when I trained regularly with weights (the reader is, perhaps, aware that for the last seven or eight years I have given my attention almost entirely to wrestling), I succeeded at St Petersburg on April 27th, 1898, in snatching 196 lb. with my right hand from the floor to above my head. This was for many years the world's record.

Approved training rules: A practice for the snatch is the lifting of a bar-bell with one hand about three feet from the floor. Snatch the weight thus up to ten times in succession to get the knack of it, for every athlete has his own personal peculiarities in lifting. By constant practice, each will find out which method of snatch is best suited to himself.

When you have managed to lift the weight above the head, make a slight turning movement to learn to hold (fix) and balance it well. In letting down the weight, use both hands.

After one has trained in this manner for four to six months—that is, having always snatched up to ten times and later increased the weight by 1 lb.—one has attained a certain agility and can try the following: Snatch the weight, which you can generally snatch ten times, thrice, increase the weight by 1 lb. to 5 lb., and snatch two or three times; then again increase by a few pounds, and snatch once or twice, and you will ascertain your own record for the time being. Between the trials, do not pause longer than one to two minutes, as otherwise the energy vanishes. It is quite sufficient to try records every three or four weeks, and in the meantime practise thoroughly exercises of endurance, and with light weights try to still improve those muscles which you have found to be somewhat flabby. It is easy to find out in what points one is lacking.

As a matter of course, all one-arm exercises are to be made right and left, so as to obtain the same strength and dexterity in both arms.

In carrying out all these exercises it is advisable to walk up and down the room continually between feats.

2. ONE-ARM SWING OF DUMB-BELL

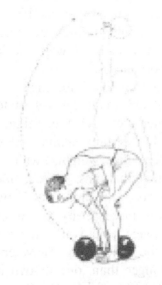

This exercise resembles the foregoing. Use a short dumb-bell.

Rule: The dumb-bell lies between the legs lengthways. The inner side of the front ball to be in line with the toes, and the weight to be raised from the floor to above the head with one movement and one arm. Some athletes stipulate that the free hand should not touch the body anywhere, and to touch the floor with the free hand would disqualify.

Execution: Seize the dumb-bell with your hand against the front ball (not in the middle), bend fairly low, and swing the weight upwards. Some athletes first swing forward to get the momentum; this is permitted.

In this performance there are the same advantages as in the snatch. French athletes excel in it.

The one-arm swing is often made with ring weights, which are swung between the legs. The Frenchman, Apollon, makes a specialty of it, and can swing four weights tied together of 180 lb. total above the head. The German, Belling, is also excellent; he swung 180 lb. three times.

As the swinging of ring weights requires a strong forearm and wrist, it is advisable to fasten a leather strap of two to three inches width round the wrist.

ONE-ARM JERK.

Rule: The weight, either bar or dumb-bell, is pushed from the shoulder to above the head with one arm, in one jerk. Whilst in England, France, and Italy it is the rule that the weight should be raised to the shoulder with one hand only, it is usual in my country (Russia) and in Germany to employ both hands. The Russian athlete Lurich, one of the best specialists in this feat, consequently raises his weight with both hands to the shoulder, and I did the same. It is, therefore, advisable to train according to the rule of one's own country or in both styles. If the weight has to be lifted to the shoulder with one arm, one may do this by snatching it or by standing the bar-bell straight up, and getting underneath it. The dumb-bell or bar-bell should, at any rate, rest free on one hand without touching the shoulder. The latter method, however, is adopted by the Austrian athletes, and they perform as a specialty the double-arm jerk of two weights in this manner. Josef Steinbach, of Vienna, one of the strongest men living, holds the world's record in the two-arm jerk of 167½ lb. and 167½ lb., both dumbbells having touched the shoulders first.

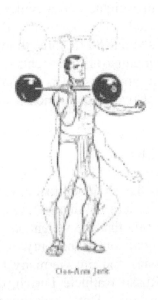

One-Arm Jerk

PRACTICAL HINTS FOR JERKING

Place the elbow of the arm, holding the weight, firmly against the body near the hip, so that the arm is somewhat relieved of the weight.

Now bend your knee slightly, and, by sudden rising and pushing upward with shoulder and arm, jerk to full arm's length above your head.

Train in the same way as indicated for the one-arm snatch.

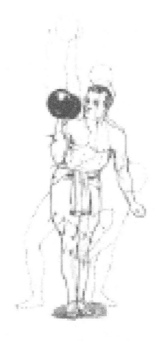

ONE-ARM PRESS

Rule: The weight, dumb-bell or bar-bell, is to be raised from the shoulder above the head without swing or jerk of the body or legs, but simply by the strength of the arms; the body may be slightly bent.

Here, also, different styles are practised in different countries in lifting the weight to the shoulders. There is a rule observed in Austria and France, but not so much in Germany, for the position of the feet during the performance, namely, the so-called " at attention " position, heels touching in military style, and pressing the weight without the slightest movement of the body. It is evident that under this rule an athlete cannot possibly press more than, say, half his own weight.

The holder of the world's record in the " at attention " position, Michael Maier, of Vienna, is especially adapted for this feat, having very short arms, and being very heavy (243 lb.) His record is 143 lb.

There have been obtained a good many noteworthy records in the ordinary one-arm press (endurance and strength feats), especially in Germany, and also in my own country (Russia). At the age of nineteen years I myself pressed a bar-bell of 269 lb. with one arm."

Arthur Saxon, the world's record holder, an athlete well known in England, has obtained wonderful results in the one-arm press. He bends himself, as it were, under the weight, and has pressed as much as 371 lb. (bar-bell) with one hand.

I may mention here that some authorities use the expression " screwing " for this kind of performance.

The real difference between " pressing " and " screwing " is, that in pressing the arm propels the weight upwards, whilst in screwing the weight hardly changes its height, as the body changes its position underneath it until the arm is stretched, after which the athlete simply erects himself. The body performance is exactly the same when you stand against a wall and press yourself away from it with one hand.

The training for the press is done in the same way as indicated for the one-arm snatch.

The so-called " screwing " is, technically, the most difficult kind of weight-lifting, and requires much practice, especially by a young athlete, whose body is still flexible. Its training should, however, be conducted very carefully, and one ought to have a friend to assist in lowering the weight, instead of letting it drop. Screwing requires a good balance of the body, and great calmness and determination. Screw as slowly as possible.

TWO-ARM SNATCH

Rule: The bar-bell is raised in one movement from floor to above the head.

This exercise, like the single-arm snatch, requires a lightning rapidity in the simultaneous working of the leg, hip, abdomen, and arm muscles; the whole body is thereby improved simultaneously, both in strength and agility.

Here also the correct exercise is the slow but gradual increase from one to five times.

TWO-ARM JERK

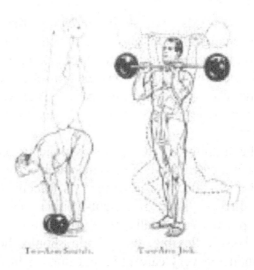

Rule: The bar-bell is pushed from the shoulder by a jerk to above the head, the legs seconding, and fixed there at least a few seconds.

This performance is, like others of which I have spoken, executed in different styles, according to the custom of the country in question. In England, France, and Italy, for instance, the bar-bell has to be raised in one movement from the floor to the shoulder, whilst in Russia, Germany, and Austria, it is permissible to raise it in several movements. Naturally, in the latter countries the results are better as far as the weight pushed is concerned. For instance, in Germany, Russia, and Austria, there are quite a number of athletes who can jerk 330 lb. and more with both arms. Josef Steinbach, of Vienna, holds the world's record with 380½ lb. I also jerked, during my training, over 330 lb.

For the French style of jerk with both arms (lifting the weight in one movement to the chest), Arvid Anderson holds the record with 328½ lb.

PRACTICAL HINTS.

The increase of the weight to lift during training is to be observed in the same gradual manner. Exercise principally in the French style (one movement to chest), which is more elegant, and is of greater value. With very heavy weights, however, lift first against the body, and then jerk up to the shoulder in one movement.

Support the weight as much as possible on the top part of the chest; do not hesitate long however, but push vigorously upwards, trying to straighten the arms as quickly as possible, and to get underneath the bar-bell. These giants' performances are only possible by the exercise of consummate technique, combined with strength. The best position of the legs is soon found out by the performer himself. Some take a step by putting one leg forward, some backward; some spread their legs much, others less. I have witnessed good results in all these positions; all depends on the individual manner.

TWO-ARM PRESS

Rule: The weight is to be raised from the shoulders above the head by the strength of the arms only, without the help of the body or legs, and fixed for a few seconds.

Here, again, the modus operandi is different in various countries. In Germany and Austria, particularly, there are a great many athletes who are very skilled in the two-arm press. This performance is technically the simplest and easiest kind of weight-lifting, as only the muscles of the shoulders and triceps are brought into play.

Training should be done in the same way as for single- arm press or push.

On the Continent, these eight styles of weight-lifting, viz., one-arm right and left snatch, jerk and press, both- arm jerk and press, are called the "Achtkampf," or the eight-lift competition, and they form, as it were, the classical test of strength. There have, however, been established records in various other forms of weight-lifting, of which I will only mention the more important ones.

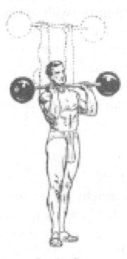

Two-Arm Press

LIFTING IN THE BRIDGE

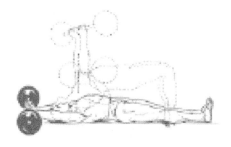

I have already recommended this exercise as excellent for the development of the spine, neck, and nape muscles, under the heading of neck muscle exercises. I will, therefore, only mention the world's record obtained by myself on August 2, 1898, in Vienna, of 311 lb. This exercise is practised principally in England, France, and Italy, where it is regarded as being the only correct style for all double-arm lifts. It forms a preliminary exercise for the double-arm snatch.

Records:—Pierre Bonnes (Paris), 330 lb.; Eliseyeff (Russia), 330 lb. I have also lifted in this style 308 lb.

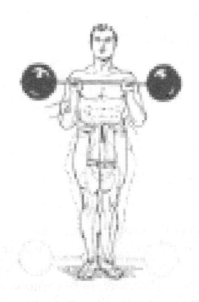

THE HORIZONTAL EQUIPOISE OF WEIGHTS

(Balancing weights with arms outstretched sideways.)

In France this performance ranks among the classical feats of strength for athletes, and there exist definite rules for its execution:—

1. The arm holding the weight to form exactly a right angle with the body, rather lower than higher.
2. The arm and wrist must be fully stretched.
3. The body must be perfectly straight, and lean in no direction.

There are two ways of performing this feat, namely—

1. The balancing of the weight on the hand, which is the less difficult.

In this case the weight is of the oblong shape used for weighing purposes, and is slightly hollowed out at the bottom, so that there is an edge. It is held so that the palm of the hand presses against this edge, while the one part of the weight rests on the wrist and the finger-tips touch the other end. One may lift the weight with both hands to the shoulder, and press it up and then let it down into the balance, or, which is considered better style, one may raise it directly sideways into the balance. It has to be fixed for a few seconds in the proper balance before being released. The weights, according to their size and heaviness, have a width from 8 to 12 in. at the bottom.

For the two-arm balance, the weights are placed with a side on the hand, so that the bottom and top of the weights are seen. In balancing, the body must not be bent backwards (which would make it easier, but which counts so many points less)

The Horizontal Equipoise, with Ring Weights

The records of this difficult performance are held by the French professional athlete Victorius, who has balanced 82½ lb. on the hand and 66 lb. by the ring.

In a less strictly correct style, I balanced on February 15, 1902, with both arms, dumb-bells of 90lb. in the right hand and 89 lb. in the left hand simultaneously, and have even held out no lb. right and 100 lb. left, simultaneously, although my performance could not be claimed as a record, seeing that it did not conform exactly to the regulations.

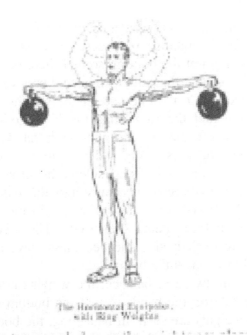

The Horizontal Equipoise with Ring Weights.

2. Balancing with ring weights is simpler in the hold, but more difficult to execute, as the palm is held downwards. The ring can, therefore, only be held against the thumb (which is more or less painful), or against the finger-ends. The weight is generally raised with slightly bent arms to the shoulders, and then held out sideways. Some prominent athletes lift it straight from the floor into the balance, and, as this is especially difficult, it counts higher.

The following are a few further records in weight-lifting and athletic performances:—

Both-arm press with two weights.

Wilhelm Turck, Vienna, on August 29, 1899: 140 lb. dumb-bell in the right hand, 139¼ lb. dumb-bell in the left hand, together 279½ lb., lifted to shoulder and correctly pressed.

The same on August 29, 1899, at Vienna: 300 lb. barbell lifted to the shoulders with both arms, and pressed.

Schneider, Cologne (Germany), 1897: 100 lb. dumbbell in each hand, twelve times.

Wilhelm Turck, Vienna, on July 30, 1901: two so-called "Boli" dumb-bells. 286 lb., correct from the shoulder to above the head.

(The lift to the shoulders was done in each case in several movements.)

Press from sitting posture (both arms).

Wilhelm Turck, on September 25, 1900: (sitting on a chair) bar-bell of 220 lb. four times, bar-bell of 237 lb. twice, bar-bell of 253 lb. once.

Lying on the floor and pulling bar-bell over the head and press.

Georg Hackenschmidt (record), August 2, 1898, in Vienna, 333 lb.

Pushing bar-bell while lying on the floor.

Georg Hackenschmidt (record), 360 lb. once (the whole body remaining on the floor).

Deep knee bending without weights.

Max Danthage, Vienna (amateur), on June 4, 1899, 6,000 times correctly within three hours.

Deep knee bending with weight on the shoulder (barbell):

H. Sell, Grossenhain (Saxony), on January 21, 1899, 440 lb. seven times; H. P. Hansen, Copenhagen, on March 19, 1899, 277 lb. sixty-five times.

Deep-knee bending, holding a bar-bell above the head with both hands.

Gustav Wain, at Reval (Russia), on January 13, 1898, 189 lb. four times.

Deep knee bend, holding a weight in each hand above the head.

G. Lurich, at Leipzig, on September 24, 1900, 110 lb. ring weight in each hand, once.

Sitting in Turkish style, and getting up with bar-bell.

George Hackenschmidt, performed at Siebert's Athletic Training School at Alsleben, Germany, in January, 1902: holding bar-bell of 187 lb. and getting up, once; holding bar-bell of no lb. and getting up, five times.

Press with the feet. (The athlete lies on his back and raises the bar-bell on the soles of the feet.)

A German amateur, Rudolf Klar, of Leipzig, has pressed in this manner 352 lb. twenty times. Arthur Saxon can support a tremendous weight on his feet in this position, probably as much as 2,500 lb.

Holding a weight (bar- or dumb-bell) with one hand erect above the head, from standing posture to lying down and getting up again.

This is an exercise which requires great strength and skill. The Swiss professional athlete, Emile Deriaz, at Paris, December, 1903, performed it with a dumb-bell of 189 lb., which he lifted first in one movement to the shoulders and pressed.

Lifting a bar-bell of 1½ in. diameter with one hand from the floor.

This performance indicates large hands and a tremendous gripping power. A Leipzig amateur thus lifted 488 lb.; it is true, only about 3½ in. from the ground. But there are athletes in Germany and Austria who can lift 420 to 440 lb. with one arm from bend to erect position of the body (hang).

Lift of bar-bell with both hands (top hold) from the floor, about six inches.

This requires great strength of arms and legs, especially strength of hips. When out of training, I lifted in Munich about 550 lb.; now a German is said to have lifted 583 lb.

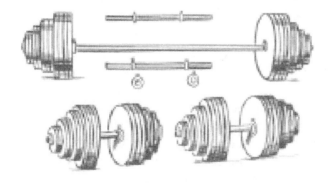

Use disc weights for preference as these are easiest altered and interchanged.

XII
TIME TABLES FOR TRAINING

IN consequence of repeated inquiries, I would here suggest a general classification of daily training, for leisured persons, invalids, etc., which may be followed or altered as individual circumstances require:—

7 a.m.—Rise, short cold rub or bath (this can be changed to tepid in winter if desired), drying preferably by exercise afterwards, but failing this by vigorous application of a rough towel. In any event, fifteen to twenty minutes' light exercises to follow the bath.

8 a.m.—Breakfast, followed by long walk till 11 a.m.

11 till 12 noon.—Vigorous exercises of any kind.

1.30 p.m.—Luncheon, and if needed, one hour's sleep to follow.

5 to 6 p.m.—Vigorous exercise for all muscles.

7.30 p.m.—Dinner, and after rest or recreation out of doors as far as possible.

11 p.m.—Bed time. (Sundays, no exercises, but a good brisk walk or walks.)

I expect that the majority of my readers, after perusing the above tables, will exclaim: "Yes, this is all very nice, and no doubt useful, but I have neither the time nor the money to live in this style."

To them, I would reply that I wished in the first instance to lay down a proper mode for training for those Physical Culture pupils whose position in life allows of their giving to it all their time for a period of a few months. If anyone should wish to excel and to become a professional athlete, he would in any case have to devote his whole time to physical culture.

Again, it might be said that no one can continue to perform these exercises every day without " knocking oneself up." To these I would reply, try it, and you will probably decide differently afterwards. Remember, though, that you must go slowly. Should your constitution to begin with be weak, unknown to you, this will be the means of improving it. Do not perform any exercises to excess, so as to tire yourself out. If you feel tired and exhausted, give yourself the necessary rest, and, as in everything else, use moderation and common sense.

Now, there are a great many people needing physical exercise, and wishing to become strong, but who lack the necessary time. I allude to people who have to work the greater part of the day. These must necessarily adapt their exercises according to circumstances.

We will, in the first instance, take the class of workers who pass most of the day behind a desk or counter, or otherwise indoors in a more or less sedentary position, or whose occupation may even bring them hurrying and flurrying through the streets. These people (supposing they have to be at their own particular work from 9 a.m. to 6 p.m., and only reach home at 7 p.m.), should extend their exercises over a longer period. They might adopt the following plan:—

Summer Time

Rise an hour before they have to leave for work, have a short cold rub or bath, then light-weight exercises as described according to muscles which specially need development, till the body dries, or if a towel be used, this should be rough and vigorously applied.

Then ordinary breakfast, and walk, instead of taking 'bus or trains, part of the way to work. In the train sit, if possible, near the open window. 7 p.m.—Good meal and rest. Afterwards vigorous exercises. 10.30 p.m.—Bed-time. Keep bedroom windows wide open in summer.

In all cases not less than eight hours' sleep.

Winter Time

Rise half an hour later than in summer, for bath, use tepid water, don't spare the towel unless the preferable mode of drying the body by exercise be adopted. Lightexercises afterwards.

Breakfast, then the same walk and manner of getting to business. Needless to say, in winter in particular, avoid draughts when you feel hot, but, otherwise, do not think that every breath of fresh air is a draught. In the evening, follow the same regime. Keep your bedroom well ventilated (during day and night), have sufficient bed-clothes, but no fires in the bedroom. Don't expose your feet to harm by the use of a warming pan or hot-water bottle.

There may be still another class of people among my readers who perform manual labor during the day for their living.

To these I particularly wish to repeat my recommendations regarding the employment of will power. They can find out which particular muscles of their body come into play during their day's work. When performing same, let me advise them, whenever possible, to put their mind into the development of these muscles, instead of working entirely mechanically. As for the development of their other muscles, they can effect this at home with the dumb-bells in the same style and manner as prescribed for this work. As their nourishment becomes sooner assimilated, they naturally require more of it; at the same time, they should also observe quite rigidly my recommendation about a good rub or bath.

In conclusion, I would like to add some general rules and reminders for observance during training, in addition to the recommendations which I have submitted at different stages of this book, and I should like my readers to

REMEMBER:

That excessive and rapid exercising is harmful.

Overwork, like laziness, spells disease.

To go ahead gently, increase your weights and exercises gradually and slowly.

That perseverance only brings permanent strength

To give their attention to all parts constituting their corporate frames, for real strength is all-round strength.

Avoid tight clothing when indoors, even dispensing with collar and coat, if practicable.

When exercising wear little or no clothes, or wear light, short, and wide knickers, and so-called gymnasium shoes.

Don't wear a tight belt.

Put sweater on during intervals, after having rubbed the perspiration off.

Avoid late suppers.

For weights, I recommend disc bells; these can be charged accurately, and do not entail the expense of many various dumb- or bar-bells of the heavier caliber.

Perform your weight-lifting in the open, if possible, otherwise on the ground floor or in a good cellar, but never on top floors.

If indoors, perform on thick planks or a thick mat. The tables for exercises mentioned should be compiled by each individual himself, according to his own judgment, based on his own observations. He must adapt them to his age and particular physical and mental constitution. My indications of weights and repetitions of the movements for each exercise will help.

And above all, remember to always walk up and down during any rest between or during exercise. Milton says: " Don't accuse nature, she has fulfilled her task; you must fulfill yours."

XII
MR von KRAJEWSKI, the FATHER OF ATHLETICS AND HIS SYSTEM OF LIFE

I HAVE previously stated that doctors, surgeons, and other medical authorities who decry rational, systematic physical exercise, and particularly, exercise with heavy weights; do so simply because they have never properly studied the subjects in question.

They may have taken a prejudice, or rather evolved a prejudice against the methods which I have ventured to style " The way to live," and having taken up this attitude, have either refused to make a personal test of them, or have not been favored with opportunities for so doing.

For the sake, therefore, of any reader who may have these prejudices, or, who may wish to combat them, I now propose to give a short sketch of a very eminent medical man, who, having his attention drawn to physical culture, at the age of forty-one, felt himself impelled to make a thorough and complete study of the subject; and also of the results of his investigation.

I shall frequently have occasion to refer to this doctor in the course of the story of my life, reference to which will show how well I was situated to form an exact observation of his daily life.

Indeed, I may say that I owe practically all that I have and am to him. He it was who taught me how to live and how to train, and he it was who launched me on my career. Would that I possessed the eloquence to express my life-long gratitude and my veneration for his memory.

Nor would I indeed claim to be his chief and only debtor. In a sense, perhaps, I owe more to him than anyone else, but athletes the world over are, one and all, directly or indirectly in his debt. Well was he styled the " Father " of athletics; for it was on the system which he first organized, that every athlete of any prominence during the last twenty-five or thirty years, developed his powers.

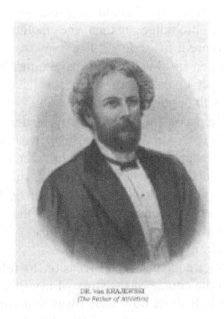

DR. von KRAJEWSKI
(The Father of Athletics)

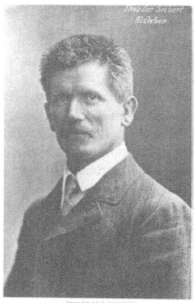

THEODORE SIEBERT

On that system and on no other, have Sandow, Saxon, Padoubny, Pierre Bonnes, Zbysco, Siegfried, Aberg, Lurich, Koch, Steinbach and hosts of others developed their powers. The doctor's system may have been varied slightly in individual cases, but the general idea, the general system and routine, nay, almost the entire programme, has in each separate instance followed closely that which Dr von Krajewski mapped out for himself.

And he, remember, was a convert. He, one of the leading physicians in St Petersburg, was attracted to the subject of physical exercise as a method of securing and preserving health, strength, activity and vigor (both mental and physical). The subject appeared interesting to him, he investigated it, approved—and immediately set to work to organize and systematize it.

First and foremost he laid it down that every man should sleep regularly for eight hours out of every twenty-four.

To this end, he would regularly, every night, on retiring to rest, write on a card the hour at which he did so; which card he would throw out into the passage, by his bedroom door. When his servant picked this up in the morning he knew at what hour the Doctor was to be called; viz., eight hours after the hour on the card, neither a moment sooner or later. Say that he had retired at four a.m. Then he would be called at noon, and so forth. Usually, however, he slept from 1 a.m. till 9 a.m., at which hour he would have coffee and rolls, and attend to his correspondence until 10 a.m.

He then adjourned to his gymnasium, a large apartment, fitted with a bath, and having two very large windows, so that as much sunlight as possible might enter. The windows, however, were never opened during the period of exercise, in order that the temperature might be as even as possible.

He would first take a short bath, in water as cold as could be obtained, and in St Petersburg the water can be cold on occasion. Leaving the bath he never used a towel, but commenced exercise straight away, and continued this for half an hour, at the end of which he would be perfectly warm and dry.

The routine followed was on the lines indicated in Chapters IX and XI (for he always exercised with weights). Naturally it would not have been possible to perform every exercise, described in these chapters, every day, but a sufficient programme was followed to bring every muscle into play, and this was so varied as to neglect none of the movements.

Between the various exercises he never sat down to rest, but walked steadily up and down the room, with perhaps a wrap thrown over his shoulders (but this rarely).

The exercise finished, he dressed and set forth on his morning round. Having visited his patients he returned home, usually about 2 p.m., for luncheon. After this he slept for one hour, and then commenced receiving patients up till 6 p.m., or thereabouts, which, with other duties, occupied him till dinner time (from seven till eight), when he resumed his attendance on indoor patients, who continued to call till as late as midnight, or even later.

This last may seem strange to British readers, but I may mention that Russian hours are much later than English ones, and that Dr Krajewski had an enormous practice, as many as 250 patients frequently calling on him in one day.

I may add that he was a most charitable man, attending numberless patients of the poorer classes without any fee or recompense. These were freely invited to call on him, and used to flock in in large numbers after 8 p.m., as they left their work; his waiting-rooms being usually crowded at that hour.

He had, of course, a large practice among the wealthy classes, which occupied the earlier part of the day.

Needless to say, such an incessant round of hard mental work and anxiety was very wearing, and would have been thought to tax the strength of even the hardiest constitution. Yet the Doctor was always well, active and vigorous in mind and body, and ascribed his perpetual fitness solely to his daily physical exercise.

As I have said, he did not commence the practice of this until he was forty-one years of age, and yet at sixty-three he always declared, and was acknowledged to look, younger, and to be far more active and vigorous than he was at forty.

So satisfied was he of the great benefits accruing from systematic physical exercise, that he spared no pains to extend its practice. His enthusiasm and interest was unbounded, while the pains which he would take to enroll adherents and to cultivate promising athletes were almost beyond belief. Some idea of these last may be gathered from a perusal of the " Story of My Life," which I have been persuaded would prove of sufficient interest to publish at length, and with which I therefore propose to conclude this book.

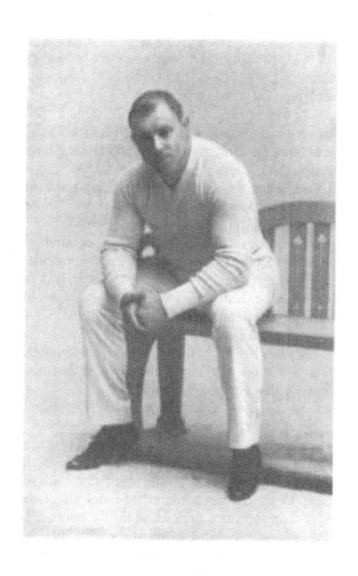

THE STORY OF MY LIFE

IT will, possibly, interest my readers to learn some details of my life and of the process of my physical development.

I was born on July 20, 1878 (Old Style), or August 2, according to English methodsof reckoning, at Dorpat in Russia, my father being the proprietor of some dye-works there. I have a brother and a sister younger than myself. Both my father and my mother were of average stature, neither of them displaying any unusual physical characteristics, but both my brother and sister possess more than average strength. My grandfather, the father of my mother—who, by the way, I never knew, as he died when I was only three years old—was always described to me as a big and powerful man. He had migrated to Russia from Sweden some sixty years before. My mother always told me that I was very like my grandfather, except that he was rather taller, being six feet in height.

So far as I can remember, I was, from my earliest years, devoted to all bodily exercises, and by the time I was eight or nine years old I used to order about a small army of boys of my own age—being admittedly the strongest of them all. I was sent to the Dorpat Grammar School (Realschule), and soon showed a preference for the hours spent in the gymnasium. At a gymnastic competition in the year 1891, when I was fourteen years old, I won a prize as the best gymnast of my own age, a fact which my instructor Herr Drewes, a German, communicated to the press in Germany. At that date, I was 4 ft 7½ in. in height and weighed 8 st. 10 lb. being of a rather thickset build. I was one of the best at club and dumb-bell exercises and could jump over 16 ft in length and 4 ft in. in height. I could raise and lower a dumb-bell weighing 1 pood (36 lb.) sixteen times with the right hand and twenty-one times with the left, and I once ran 180 metres (about 197 yards) in 26 seconds.

My liking for bodily exercises I inherited from my grandfather.

On leaving school in 1895, I entered some large engineering works in Reval as an apprentice, with a view to becoming a practical and technical engineer. But— Man proposes, God disposes!

At this time I became a member of the Reval Athletic and Cycling Club, and threw myself heart and soul into cycling, at which I won several prizes.

When autumn and bad weather came round, I gave more attention to exercises with heavy weights and dumbbells and my ambition soon led me to excel all my fellow members in these exercises.

The chief pastimes favored in our club were the lifting of heavy weights and wrestling. For the latter I had at first but little liking and was often beaten.

About this time I grew pretty quickly, my measurements in 1896, at the age of eighteen, being as follows:— Height . . 5 ft 7½ in. Chest . . 41½ in. normal and 44 in. expanded. Biceps. . 14 in. straight and 15½ in. flexed. Forearm . 12½ in.

We had a very judicious trainer in our club, a certain Gospodin (Mr) Andruschkewitsch, a government official, who gave us young fellows many excellent hints on the care and training of the body. At a Club festival held about this time (autumn of 1896) I performed the following weight-lifting feats:—

With the right hand from the shoulder I pressed 145 lb. 12 times, 155 lb. 10 times, 198 lb. 3 times, 214 lb. 1 time and with one hand lifting slowly from the ground to the shoulder (by the strength of the biceps) I raised a weight of 125 lb. with the right, and of 119 lb. with the left.

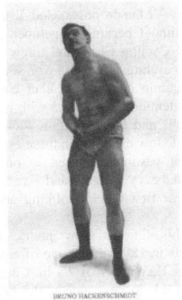

BRUNO HACKENSCHMIDT
Hackenschmidt's brother

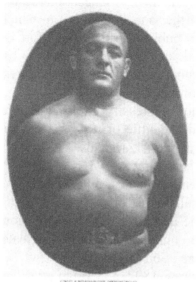

CYGANIEWICZ ZBYSZKO

In September, 1896, I made the acquaintance of the professional athlete and wrestler, Lurich. He was only a few years older than myself, had been a professional for a year, and was touring in the Eastern Provinces with a small company.

Lurich challenged all comers to wrestle with him and various members of our club came forward but were all, without exception, defeated by him. Up to this time, I had shown but little taste for wrestling and had wrestled very seldom, being more partial to work with heavy weights. Still, I wrestled several times with Lurich, who, even then, was a fairly good wrestler, though, as I speedily recognized, scarcely my equal in strength. As can readily be understood, Lurich had no great difficulty in throwing an inexperienced man, such as I was, though on the one occasion on which I wrestled with him in public—in the Standpfort Etablissement in Reval—he could not throw me the first time, and in the second bout I was able to resist him for seventeen minutes.

I mention this easily intelligible defeat, incurred when I had had little or no experience in wrestling, because, later on, Lurich used to boast that he had frequently beaten me.

This gentleman has, since then, for many years kept carefully out of my way, but this defeat annoyed me and after it I wrestled more frequently and, in the course of the winter, defeated nearly all the members of our club.

In February, 1897, a German wrestler, Fritz Konietzko came to Reval. It was said that at Magdeburg he had beaten the famous Tom Cannon, then in his prime, who, in his day, had often wrestled with Abs, a wrestler who enjoyed a big reputation in Germany, and had thus achieved some celebrity in the Graeco-Roman style. Konietzko was a rather smaller man than myself, being 5 ft in. in height and barely turning the scale at 165 lb. Taking him all round his was not a very imposing figure. Yet he was very quick and possessed a strength of hand which to me seemed almost uncanny. These qualities enabled him to defeat all his opponents; especially as he was always undermatched. I was the only member of the amateur contingent to withstand the German. We wrestled ten minutes without a fall. Not long after this Ladislaus Pytlasinski, the Polish wrestler, then at the zenith of his fame, came to Reval and, of course, defeated Konietzko. Pytlasinski defeated me easily, and we all learnt a great deal from this great expert of the wrestling arena. In the following year he was the first wrestler to defeat the famous Turk, Kara Ahmed in Paris. I remember, too, a very powerful village schoolmaster in the neighborhood of Reval who was one of the chief opponents of this professional wrestler. He (the schoolmaster) had only a few holds, with which he defeated his opponents. On one occasion he got me down in seven minutes.

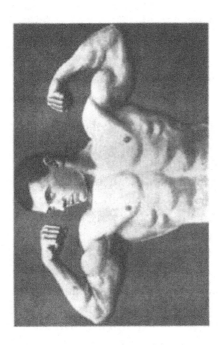

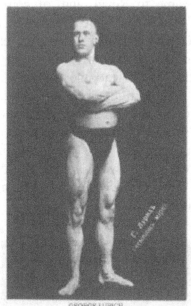

GEORGE LURICH

As I have said already, these defeats proved very instructive to me and I gradually, if slowly, began to perfect myself in wrestling.

I improved rapidly in lifting power and also in general physical development, and by July, 1897, I was able to press a bar weighing 243 lb. with both hands from my shoulders to the full stretch of my arms. Even at this date I established a world's record—which was, of course, very soon broken, but afterwards improved on, and since maintained by myself. With my hands crossed behind my back and my knees bent, I lifted a ball weighing 171 lb. This feat proved that I was fairly strong in the legs. Taking two balls weighing 94½ lb. each in either hand, I swung them with a single motion from the ground to the full stretch of the arms. Our instructor, Gospodin Andruschkewitz, took my measurements in December, 1897, with the following results:—

Height	5 ft. 8½ in.
Neck	18¼ in.
Biceps	15¾ in. straight, and 17¼ flexed.
Forearm	13 in.
Wrist	7½ in.
Chest	44⅞ in. normal and 46 in. expanded.
Thigh	23½ in.
Calf	15⅓ in.
Weight	12 st. 8 lb.

In December, 1897, I performed the following feats:—

Jerked up a bar of 216 lb. twelve times with both hands.

Jerked up a bar of 187 lb. seven times with one hand.

Pressed up a bar of 216 lb. with one hand.

About this time I was thrown in contact with a remarkable man, who exercised a notable influence on my future life.

A slight injury sustained in the exercise of my calling as an engineer—for I was still an amateur—made it necessary for me to seek the help of a doctor. This doctor, an amiable old gentleman, happened to have staying with him a distinguished colleague, Dr von Krajewski, a physician in ordinary to His Majesty the Czar. This Dr von

Krajewski was the founder of the St Petersburg Athletic and Cycling Club, of which H.R.H. the Grand Duke Vladimir Alexandrovitch was President, and which included many aristocratic and wealthy people among its members. Dr Krajewski, in spite of his fifty-six years, was still a very active and energetic man, and particularly keen on feats of strength and weight-lifting. He had first taken up this pastime at the mature age of forty-one, and by systematic training had attained to a fairly high degree of physical strength. The doctor had, of course, visited our club and recognized me at once. When I had completely undressed in order to facilitate a careful examination of my injury, he, in conjunction with my own doctor, examined my body, and found that with the exception of a slight injury (a contusion of the arm) I was perfectly sound. He invited me to come and stay with him in St Petersburg as he wished to have me trained as a professional athlete and wrestler.

I learned that Dr von Krajewski had also had Lurich in training with him for some time, and he was good enough to say that I possessed possibilities of becoming the strongest man in the world.

Yielding to the persuasion of all my club friends, who congratulated me warmly on Dr von Krajewski's offer, but against the wishes of my parents, I set out for St Petersburg early in 1898.

Dr von Krajewski was a bachelor and lived in a large house in the Michael Platz, St Petersburg. He had an excellent practice in the highest circles of society and passed for a millionaire. I was most hospitably received in the house of this patron of athletics. The doctor treated me like a son and gave me the best training his experience could suggest. One room in his house was hung with portraits of all the best-known strong men and wrestlers, and he delighted in inviting them to his house, in which all foreign artistes found hospitable welcome every month. Dr von Krajewski was the organizer of a private club of men of fashion who came to him weekly and worked hard with weights and dumbbells, and practised wrestling. In his gymnasium the doctor had a great number and variety of weights, dumb-bells, and other apparatus and appliances for the purposes of training. It was, in short, a fully equipped school of physical culture.

All the professional strong men and wrestlers who appeared at the St Petersburg theatres visited Dr von Krajewski and gave exhibitions of their art. While so doing, they were all carefully examined, measured and weighed. Dr von Krajewski had thus been able to acquire great experience and knowledge of feats of strength and methods of training.

The example set by these artistes had a most stimulating influence on us all. Everyone seemed put upon his mettle to do his very best. Having now nothing to occupy me but alternate exercise and rest, I made rapid progress in strength. The doctor told me not to touch alcoholic drinks and tobacco, for neither of which I had ever felt any great inclination, and in neither of which I had ever indulged.

I drank little else but milk (3 litres, or more than 11 pints daily) and ate practically what I pleased, my appetite being then, as always, an excellent one. I bathed daily with the Doctor in his bath-room, a very spacious apartment built in close proximity to the gymnasium. After the bath we practised weight-lifting till we got dry, neither of us using the towel to dry ourselves. In January, 1898, I pushed up a bar weighing 275 lb. to the full height of the arms, and with the right hand pushed up 243 lb., and lying on the ground, I lifted and pushed up with two hands a weight of 304 lb., following this soon after with one of 335 lb. With the knees bent I raised a weight of 108½ lb., which remained a world's record for many years till beaten by me with 187 lb. in 1902.

In February I accompanied Dr von Krajewski to Moscow, where Baron Kister, another great patron of athletics, had organized a weight-lifting competition for amateurs. I was fairly successful here, and managed to raise a weight of 255½ lb. with one hand. For this feat I was soon after my return awarded a gold medal by my club, the St Petersburg Athletic and Cycling Club, of which I had become a member. The training at Dr von Krajewski's was very many-sided and I rapidly gained strength in all parts of the body. I also trained steadily in wrestling, the frequent visits of professional wrestlers to the doctor's house affording me many excellent opportunities. About this time Count Ribeaupierre, Master of the Horse to H.M. the Czar, became President of the St Petersburg Athletic and Cycling Club.

This gentleman took a keen interest in me and has continued to manifest his good will towards me ever since. He afterwards frequently supported and helped me, and I feel that I owe him a debt of gratitude.

In April, 1898, my club organized a weightlifting competition for the championship of Russia, in which I won first prize and accomplished the following among other feats.

With both hands I lifted 114 kilogrammes or 251 lb. to full height of arms with a jerk (being only 1 kilogramme less than the world's record of the Frenchman, Bonnes— 115 kilogrammes).

I snatched up 257 lb. with both hands.
With the right hand jerked 231 lb.
With the left hand jerked 205 lb.
With the right hand pressed 269 lb.

Towards the end of April the famous French wrestler Paul Pons came to St Petersburg, and I defeated this practised wrestler at the end of forty-five minutes. I also threw Jankowsky in eleven minutes. It is possible that Pons may not have been in his best form on this occasion, as he himself maintained, for some time afterwards I had a much tougher struggle with him.

I was in tip-top condition and was continuing to train steadily when Dr von Krajewski put down my name to contest the championship of the world and the championship of Europe at the end of July and beginning of August which were to be wrestled for in connection with the Sports Exhibition in Vienna.

In order to accustom myself to appearing before large audiences, I performed for some weeks previously in a circus at Riga, as an athlete and wrestler, under an assumed name. Dr von Krajewski, who had an eye for everything, did not omit to take into account the embarrassment which a young performer is certain to feel when he first faces a large audience. I earned a good deal of applause and threw all opponents in wrestling. But to be quite candid, even at that time I still possessed but little of the technique of wrestling. I was, however, very strong and took all my opponents unawares in a few minutes. Even my former conqueror, Kalde, the teacher already mentioned, was obliged to admit this, as I threw the good man repeatedly after very short struggles, at which he was not a little surprised. Before we set out for Vienna, Dr von Krajewski took careful measurements of me, with the following results:—

Height	5 ft. $9\frac{1}{2}$ in.
Weight	14 st.
Waist	$32\frac{3}{4}$ in.
Neck	$18\frac{1}{4}$ in.
Chest and shoulders	$47\frac{1}{4}$ in. normal and 51 in. expanded.
Right shoulder joint	$21\frac{5}{8}$ in.
Left shoulder joint	$21\frac{1}{2}$ in.
Biceps of right arm	$15\frac{1}{4}$ in. $16\frac{3}{4}$ in.
Biceps of left arm	$14\frac{7}{8}$ in. $16\frac{1}{2}$ in.
(measured when flexed and straight)	
Forearm, right	$13\frac{5}{8}$ in.
Forearm, left	$13\frac{1}{4}$ in.
Right and left wrist	$7\frac{3}{4}$ in.
Right and left thigh	$24\frac{1}{4}$ in.
Calf	$15\frac{1}{4}$ in.
Ankle	$9\frac{1}{8}$ in.

My best performances, at the end of the six months which I spent with the hospitable doctor, in addition to those already mentioned were as follows:—

I jerked a bar weighing 306 lb. with both hands.

I pulled in clean to the shoulders a bar weighing 361 lb.

I snatched a bar weighing 197½ lb. with the right hand (a world's record).

These feats were performed either in the Doctor's gymnasium or in Count Ribeaupierre's riding school and the weights were in every instance carefully checked. This reminds me of a humorous incident over which I have often laughed heartily. The doctor was at this time wearing a new pair of trousers, which fitted him exceedingly well, insomuch that I more than once expressed a wish to possess similar garments. Dr von Krajewski jestingly replied, " My dear George, when you can beat Sandow's world's record of putting up 116 kilogrammes or 255½ lb. with one hand you shall have just such another pair! " It may have been this jest which spurred me on to make a special effort by pulling up a weight of 122.25 kilogrammes (269½ lb. English). This was done in Count Ribeaupierre's private riding school, which was arranged for this occasion like a circus. The place was filled with a large audience of some of the most distinguished people in St Petersburg. When I lifted this weight Dr Krajewski in front of all the people rose from his seat, and lifted his hat to full arm's length above his head. I shall never forget the doctor on this occasion. His admiration for feats of strength was almost beyond understanding.

Everybody was surprised by this evidence of his genuine emotion, and it seemed as though his enthusiasm spread itself over the whole of the audience, everybody congratulating me warmly. The doctor disappeared for a few minutes and returned with the promised pair of trousers. I don't mind admitting that, at the moment, I was almost more pleased with this gift than with the large gold Record Medal solemnly presented to me a few days later.

There was, indeed, something singular, I had almost said something mysterious, about Dr von Krajewski. Something in the man's being seemed to melt in his love for feats of strength and agility, and flowed forth in an inexplicable fire on all artistes of this genre. These people often used to say to me, " We don't know how it is, but once the doctor appears on the scene one feels as though one had more strength." This was just the feeling I always had, but it surprised me to hear my impression confirmed by others. I went to Vienna in company with Dr von Krajewski, and the pick of the St Petersburg amateurs, Guido Meyer and Alexander von Schmelling. We were most hospitably received by the Vienna Athletic Club, and I made the acquaintance of various first-rate athletes and wrestlers.

It was there I first met Wilhelm Turck, a very strong man, at that time about forty years of age. He is nearly 6 ft high and weighs 18 st. 12 lb. He could raise, largely by main force, a bar weighing 330 lb. to the full height of his arms, and could draw up a weight of 132 lb. in both hands simultaneously (264 lb. in all). My best performance at that time was 114 lb. in each hand, or 228 lb. in all. But in putting up a weight with one hand, which requires more skill, he could only manage 138½ lb. as against my 242 lb.

I may here point out that owing to the excitement attendant on such events it is very difficult for a man to do his best. My performances were:—

Jerking a bar with both hands, 311 lb.
Slow pressing a bar with both hands, 249 lb.
Slow pressing a bar with both hands, 220 lb., four times.

In weight-lifting I was third, behind Turck and Binder, the latter also a Viennese athlete.

It seemed to me that the arrangement of the contests was all in favor of the Viennese, for even the very strong French champion, Pierre Bonnes, could not win a place, owing to the fact that the Viennese had, undoubtedly, been exclusively trained for these special feats. The same remark applies to the feats with separate weights (i.e., with the so-called short Bohlig dumb-bells). My fellow clubman, Meyer, it is true, made a very creditable show, but even he could not score much. Herr von Schmelling, a very tall man, 6 ft 4½ in. in height and about 17 st. 4 lb. in weight, had wrestled with me and with Paul Pons for a full hour without decisive result, and was reckoned a better wrestler than I, but he had very poor luck in Vienna, for, after defeating Wetasa, the best Viennese wrestler of that day, after a contest of one and half hours, he had, owing to a misunderstanding with the umpire, to retire from a second contest with Burghardt. I was now Dr von Krajewski's sole remaining hope in the wrestling bouts. I was in excellent fettle, and, first of all, threw several Viennese amateurs in very quick time, less than one minute each. I was then matched with the Bavarian champion, Michael Hitzler, a wonderfully good wrestler, but rather too light a weight for me. I put out my full force and threw him after a plucky struggle lasting five minutes. It took me only two minutes to settle with Burghardt, who was not so good a man.

I had now won the first prize in wrestling, the championship of Europe, a beautiful gold medal, and a magnificent championship-belt. Dr von Krajewski was delighted, and congratulations rained down on me from every side. Professor Hueppe of Prague was one of the umpires in this competition. An enthusiast in gymnastics, he took a great interest in the wrestling contests and was good enough to praise me very highly. I received quite a general ovation at the supper given at the close of the contest, and the Athletic Club invited Dr von Krajewski, Meyer, von Schmelling and myself to a soiree.

Towards evening on the following day we found ourselves in the Club rooms, and the old doctor was the first to make himself at home and laid hold of the tools. Great surprise was shown on every side at seeing so old a man so keen at his work. He put up a bar of 154 lb. several times with two hands and performed a number of other feats of strength. Fired by his example, I achieved the following performance: lying on the ground I raised above the head and put up 331½ lbs.

Next day, on the invitation of one of the umpires, Herr Victor Silberer, we made an excursion to this gentleman's country house on the Semmering Pass, and spent a most enjoyable time. Herr Silberer is the proprietor and editor of the Allgemeine Sport Zeitung, and himself a keen sportsman. After our return to St Petersburg I was challenged on various pretexts by Wetasa of Vienna, and also by Lurich to wrestle for the championship of Europe or to defend the same. Dr von Krajewski undertook the preliminaries, but both men sought to insist on such impossible conditions that the contest fell through. Even at that date I had not the slightest fear of either of them. Wetasa was already somewhat past his prime, while I knew that Lurich, though somewhat more experienced, was a weaker wrestler than myself. I spent the remainder of the year at Dr von Krajewski's, and in January, 1899, after a keen struggle won the championship of Finland from twenty competitors.

Although from the date of my first great success in the wrestling ring onwards I trained less and less for weight- lifting records, yet in January, 1899, I pressed a bar of 279½ lb. with both hands.

The time for my enrolment in the army had now arrived, and I was commanded to join the Preobrashensky Polk (the 1st Life Guards of the Tsar), but was released from service after five months. On May 16, in Count Ribeaupierre's riding school, I wrestled to a finish the contest with Herr von Schmelling which had been left undecided in the previous year and defeated him in twenty-five minutes by means of a " half-nelson," thus winning the championship for 1898. A few days later, on May 19, a second victory over Schmelling in forty-four minutes gained me the Russian championship for 1899. Schmelling was one of my toughest opponents!

After this, I again trained for some time at weight- lifting and made some progress, as I jerked a bar of 330 lb. with both hands, but in trying to slow press 286 lb. with one hand, I strained a sinew in my right shoulder, an injury which was destined to trouble me for years afterwards. At first I thought little of this trifling pain and trained for the Championship of the World wrestling contests in Paris, which took place in November. I was firmly resolved to become a professional wrestler. Although my arm had not yet fully recovered I went to Paris and took part in the contests.

The list of competitors for this tournament was as follows: Charles le Meunier (France), Henri Pechon (France), Francois le Farinier (Swiss), Feriol Marius (France), Henri Alphonse (Swiss), Loirdit Porthos, Trillat le Savoyard, Capitant le Parisien, Louis Chappe (all of France), Niemann (Germany), Camillus Evertsen (Denmark), Pietro Dalmasso (Italy), Barnet le Demenageur (France), Jaccavail (France), Devaux (Belgium), Dirk van den Berg (Holland), Raoul le Boucher (France), Raymond Franc (France), Victor Delmas (France), Edgar Joly (France), Hautier le Breton, Leon le Jouteur (France), Bonera Domenico (Italy), Aimable de la Calmette (France), Starck

(Germany), Jean le Marseil- lais (France), Edouard Robin (France), Jax le Taureau (France), Henri Lorange (France), Fengler (Germany), Alis-Amba (Africa), Eberle (Germany), Robinet (France), Laurent le Beaucairois (France), Constant le Boucher (Belgium), Kara Ahmed (Turkey), Peyrousse (France), Charles Poiree (France), Miller (Germany), Paul Pons (France), besides myself.

My first opponent was a medium wrestler, Loir, nicknamed Porthos. I got him down in eighteen seconds! My second was a Frenchman from the South, named Robinet, a wrestler with a fairly good style and till then of fairly high reputation. It is, perhaps, only natural that foreign wrestlers should be greeted with a certain amount of distrust. I was at that time almost unknown to the general public in France, and everyone was astonished to see me defeat the popular Robinet in the short space of four minutes. Robinet was too sportsmanlike to attribute his defeat to accident, but, in answer to questions, said that I was very strong; "he has a grip like a vice, and if he gets you on the ground you are done for." It was about this time that people began to call me " the Russian Lion."

After the struggle with Robinet, the next morning I went to the Gymnasium Piaza, Rue Faubourg St Denis, to train, when Leon Dumont, the French wrestler, put my shoulder out of joint, and for a long time my right arm seemed half paralysed. Monsieur Piaza used hot and cold shower-baths and electricity to try to restore the use of my arm, but with little result.

It has long been the custom in wrestling circles to put all sorts of difficulties in the way of beginners who threaten to prove dangerous rivals later on, and thus to scare the newcomers out of the profession. I myself was told that " Beginners who may become dangerous must be defeated often and severely in order to get rid of them."

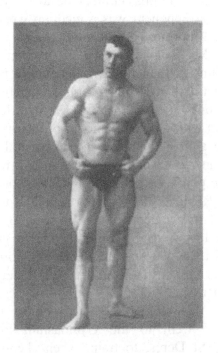

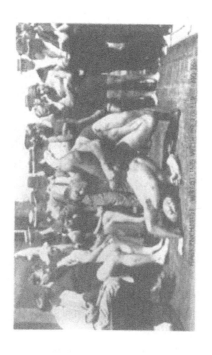

In accordance with this policy the third opponent assigned to me was one of the best French wrestlers, the versatile Aimable de la Calmette. This athlete, as I soon discovered, was not nearly so strong as I, but far more experienced, a fact which made it necessary for me to be careful, for an experienced wrestler is far more dangerous than one who is merely strong. One is never safe from surprises, and it is almost impossible to calculate on what such wrestlers may do. Well, I threw the worthy Aimable after forty-seven minutes, but learned a great deal in the course of this struggle. On the following day Laurent le Beaucairois, a very strong and clever performer, appeared upon the scene. Till then I had not believed it possible that so corpulent a man—Laurent weighed 18 st. 12 lb., though he was slightl y shorter than I —could show so much activity and nimbleness. Laurent was an old hand at the game, having wrestled for fifteen years, and it did not look as if there was much chance for me who had scarcely had fifteen months' experience. In strength I was the Frenchman's equal, if not his superior, and I made up my mind to be on my guard and give no chances. We wrestled for thirty minutes when the referee declared the contest a draw.

After this last bout the weakness in my arm gave me a good deal of trouble, and I thought it best to retire from the tournament, especially as a French surgeon had ordered me to avoid all overstraining for twelve months. I sincerely wish that I had followed his advice!

I looked on at a few more contests and then returned home to have my arm seen to, going in for treatment with electricity for about six months, but I am inclined to fancy that this did me more harm than good. All went well, and in May, 1900, I again began to lift heavy weights.

With the thoughtlessness of youth, I soon began to lift the heaviest bars again, and my arm, which had scarcely recovered, was again injured in an attempt to establish fresh records in weight-lifting. Dr von Krajewski warned me seriously, and I grew more prudent and avoided tours de force of this nature

In June, 1900, a wrestling combat took place at Moscow. This was my first appearance as a professional wrestler. The tournament lasted forty days, my salary being 2,500 francs (or £100) per month. We were wrestling for two prizes, viz., the Championships of St Petersburg and of Moscow. As I succeeded in winning both I gained another 1,500 fr. for the St Petersburg championship and 2,500 fr. more, being the amount of the first Moscow prize. I met Aimable and Petroff, and defeated them. I also threw the eel-like Constant le Boucher, a young Belgian, in five minutes. Petroff was an immensely strong Bulgarian. Constant was incredibly clever and agile, but seemed to undervalue me as an opponent. As he admitted afterwards, he had heard me described as being somewhat clumsy, though very strong. After defeating Constant, the French wrestlers put Peyrousse forward against me. This wrestler was tremendously powerful, but had little heart, so that hardly had we commenced struggling than he practically threw himself, greatly to the surprise of his compatriots, who had counted on his crushing me. My second bout with him lasted only seven seconds. Following Peyrousse I met and defeated an enormously strong Cossack in Michailoff, whom I threw in ten minutes. While our championship matches in Moscow were still proceeding a great wrestling competition had already commenced in Vienna. Unfortunately I entered too late and did not reach Vienna until the final stages were in progress. My old opponent Pons took first prize. Kara Ahmed, a first-rate Turkish wrestler, was second, and the corpulent Laurent third. Neither Pons nor the Turk would consent to meet me. Apparently they were in no hurry to risk their freshly-won laurels. The good-natured Laurent alone was willing to wrestle a fall with me. I first of all had a bout with a very tall and heavy Spaniard, named Chorella, whom I threw in the short space of twenty-nine seconds. I had more trouble with a Dutchman, Dirk van den Berg, a finely built athlete. Van den Berg played a defensive game, looking out for some oversight on my part, but at length I defeated him in twenty- two minutes. I found an even more wily opponent in the German Fengler, who seemed a good-natured man and made all sorts of proposals to me before the contest, but once we set to work I found that he was only too anxious to beat me. I now began to realize that in order to win one requires not only brute strength, but must also employ in a far greater degree than the uninitiated would suppose, both judgment and reflection. I threw Fengler in twenty-six minutes. On the next day I wrestled with the doughty and corpulent Laurent le Beaucairois. We had a pretty lively set-to, and the Frenchman let it clearly be seen that he had no hope of beating me, for at the end of an hour he withdrew from the contest. Early in September I went to Dresden, the capital of Saxony, to attend a small wrestling competition. I was the chief attraction there, and wrestled almost nightly with from three to five opponents, nearly all of whom I defeated very quickly, e.g.:—

Winzer of Hamburg in seven minutes, The Austrian Burghardt in six minutes, And the two nimble Italian brothers, Emilio and Giovanni Raicevieh, in three and six minutes respectively, all in a single evening! I threw Fengler and Konietzko on another evening in three minutes altogether. At Dresden I met a very stout and heavy wrestler named Sebastian Miller. This worthy man weighed nearly 24 st., and was fairly strong, but so deficient in science that I threw him in three minutes, and immediately afterwards a nimble but smaller Frenchman named Maurice Gambier in five minutes, and Hitzler in twenty-three minutes. Hitzler had improved greatly. I took the first prize at Dresden.

From Dresden I went to Chemnitz, another Saxon town of somewhat less than a quarter of a million inhabitants. Here the contestants were: Gambier (France), Hofer (Germany), Seb Miller (Germany), Konietzko (Germany), Buisson (France), Hitzler (Germany), Winzer (Germany), Giovanni and Emilio Raicevich (Italy), Rossner (Germany), Petri (Holland), Oscar Uhlig (Germany), Burghardt (Austria), Diriks (Belgium) and myself. At Chemnitz I, for the first time, met my old antagonist Lurich. As often happens, the management of another theatre, in order to compete with our undertaking, had engaged Lurich and a number of other inferior wrestlers. Lurich went about boasting loudly that he had more than once defeated me with ease. His impresario billed Lurich as the strongest man in the world and " the invincible wrestler."

Though as a rule I have no great liking for impromptu challenges, yet in view of this continuous and brazen puffing of Lurich I could not refrain from challenging him to a wrestling match, when I found that he persisted in these wanton personal attacks upon me. Accordingly Hitzler and I strolledround one evening—it was Monday, September 17—to the theatre at which Lurich was engaged and offered to wrestle with him. Although Lurich had declared himself ready to meet any wrestler, amateur or professional, who chose to come forward, our challenge was not accepted, on the plea that the " invincible " had already his full quota of opponents. It was nevertheless announced from the stage that Herr Lurich would wrestle with Hackenschmidt on the following Wednesday. On the appointed evening we were punctually in our places, but we noticed that Lurich was already provided with two opponents. One of these, who seemed to be quite ignorant of wrestling, he threw in less than a minute. He then prepared to serve his second opponent in similar fashion when this latter suddenly vanished from the stage, crying out as he went, " Yonder stands Herr Hackenschmidt" (pointing at me), "he will take my place, as I don't feel well." I went on to the stage, amid thunderous applause from the crowded audience which had assembled, in order to wrestle with Lurich. But no sooner did the " invincible wrestler" catch sight of me than he turned deadly pale and bolted into the wings, and in spite of repeated calls he absolutely declined to return. The Chemnitz Allgemeine Zeitung (No. 29, of September 21, 1900) printed the following note on this incident:—

" As our readers are aware, George Lurich, who describes himself as the ' Champion Athlete of the World' and ' Strongest Man in the World,' has for some days past been appearing at the Mosella Saal. In addition to a somewhat glowing advertisement of his powers, he has issued on his bills, etc., etc., a challenge to all wrestlers, whether amateur or professional. On Monday evening George Hackenschmidt, who is taking part in a wrestling competition at the Kaufmannische Vereinshaus, challenged him to a wrestling bout on Wednesday evening. News of this spread very quickly among all the sporting elements of Chemnitz, with the result that the Mosella Saal was packed from floor to ceiling on the evening in question. Everyone looked forward with impatience for the beginning of the wrestling match. The disappointment of the spectators can therefore be imagined, when Herr Lurich appeared on the stage in the company of Herr Gleissner of Borna and another gentleman of whose identity we are ignorant. To dispose of a wrestler like Herr Gleissner was, of course, mere child's play for Herr Lurich. The second wrestler retired in favour of Herr Hackenschmidt, whose challenge had been given on Monday evening, and who therefore had the prior claim. Hereupon the curtain was abruptly lowered amid stormy scenes on the part of the indignant audience. Cries of ' Come out! ' ' Shame ! ' ' Swindle ! ' were quickly heard, mingled with whistling and cat-calls enough to make one's flesh creep. All this was directed against the ' invincible' Herr Lurich, who, we are informed, has caused similar scandals in other towns, such as Elberfeld, where the competitors in the International Wrestling Contests were unfortunately prevented by the terms of their engagement from exposing the Russian in the manner adopted on Wednesday. Even the management of the Mosella Saal failed to persuade Lurich to meet Hackenschmidt. Presumably Lurich will not be allowed to appear again until he has wrestled with Hackenschmidt, who is ready to meet him on any evening."

Lurich left Chemnitz on the following morning.

My sole object in recording this unpleasant incident is to enable the English public to estimate at their true value the insinuations directed against me by a fellow countryman in the summer of 1904. We continued our tournament at Chemnitz undisturbed, and in addition to winning first prize I received a splendid ovation from the public. Hitzler and Gambier gaining second and third prizes respectively.

From Chemnitz I journeyed to Buda Pesth, the beautiful capital of Hungary, where a wrestling contest had commenced on September 24. The participants were: Kara Ahmed (Turkey), Robinet (France), Muldoon (of America, but not the celebrated Physical Culturist), Charles (France), Krendel (Austria), Weber (Germany), Hitzler (Germany), Celestin Moret (France), Lassartesse (France), Ignace Nollys (Belgium), Albert de Paris (France), Giovanni Raicevich (Italy), Pibius (France), Burghardt (Austria), Mayer (Hungary), and Sandorfi (Hungary), Aimable (France), etc.

One of my first opponents was Robinet, who was a great favourite with the Buda Pesth public, on the strength of his performances some years previously. I threw the Frenchman in eight minutes, and, later on in the competition, I defeated Albert de Paris, a very clever wrestler, in five minutes, Weber, of Germany, in two minutes, Aimable in twenty-five minutes, and Van den Berg in twenty- four minutes. My severest bout was with the Turk, Kara Ahmed, whom it took me nearly three hours to defeat. But never, while I live, shall I forget what then took place. The whole audience rose like one man, and thunders of applause echoed through the building. I was seized, carried shoulder high, and decked with flowers. For fully a quarter of an hour I was borne like a victorious general through the streets, kissed, embraced, etc., etc. I can assure you I was heartily glad when I at last made my escape to the privacy of the dressing-room. Never, even in Paris, have I experienced a similar ovation. I am not likely to forget those worthy Hungarians. The result was as follows. I won the first prize of 1,500 kronen besides my salary, the second prize of 1,000 kronen going to Kara Ahmed, and the third of 600 kronen to Dirk van den Berg, and the fourth of 400 kronen to Aimable de la Calmette.

We left the hospitable walls of Buda Pesth, and I next won the first prize at Graz, in Steiermark. None of the contests there were of great importance. At Graz I was pitted against the German athlete Rasso, an exceedingly powerful man, but no wrestler. I threw him as I pleased, clean and cleverly in five minutes, to the great surprise of the good people of Graz, who were familiar with Rasso's Herculean feats as an athlete.

Towards the end of October, I gained a first prize at Nurnberg, a prominent city of Bavaria, after which I returned to St Petersburg, as my arm had again become almost useless owing to the continual strain to which it had been subjected. After eight weeks' rest, during which my arm underwent thorough treatment, my ambition again drove me to Paris in order to wrestle matches with Pons, Beaucairois, Constant, Van den Berg, and Aimable. I twice defeated Aimable, once in thirty-four and once in seventeen minutes. Van den Berg I threw in twenty-five and in three minutes. My first bout with Constant lasted an hour without result, and then we wrestled for two hours and a quarter, when he was declared the loser. Pons avoided meeting me. But Beaucairois, who must have known that I was suffering from a sharp attack of influenza, ventured to try his luck with me. I defeated him in twenty minutes, and then, in spite of my ailing condition, wrestled for an hour without result, and at the end of the day, in defiance of my doctor's advice, I again began to wrestle with the doughty Laurent. Half unconscious owing to the fever which coursed through my veins, after a struggle of twenty-three minutes, I fell a victim to a bras roule of the Frenchman's. This was, strictly speaking, the first fall I had incurred in the course of my otherwise victorious career as a professional wrestler, and it was entirely due to my pride, since the Paris doctor called it inexcusable on my part to think of wrestling in such a condition!

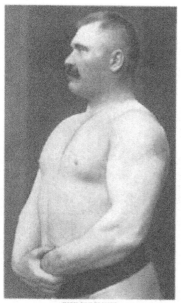
IVAN PADOUBNY

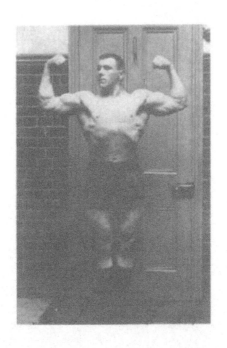

I had scarcely recovered when I had to fulfill an engagement in Hamburg, where the following wrestlers were engaged in a tournament: Max Nitsche (Berlin), Strenge Berlin), Tom Clayton—" Bulldog(England), Joe Carroll (England), Lassartesse (France), Branken (Holland), Giovanni Raicevich (Italy), Celestin Moret (France), Weber (Germany), Saurer (Bavaria), G. Lurich (Russia), Pietro le Beige (Belgium), G. Semmel (Hamburg), Constant le Boucher (Belgium), G. Jeurisson (Belgium), Emil Bau (Germany), H. Landy (Holland), H. Oehlers (Hamburg) Kara Mustapha (Turkey), Clement le Terrassier (Belgium), Hitzler (Bavaria), Poiree (France), Kreindl (Austria), Peyrousse (France), JessPedersen (Denmark),

Lemmertz (Germany), Winzer (Hamburg), Hassan Omer (Turkey), Orondi (Steiermark), Dirk van den Berg (Holland), Diriks (Belgium), P. Belling (Berlin), H. Eberle (Germany) and Halil Adali, undoubtedly the best wrestler Turkey has ever produced. I first wrestled with some less important men, and then beat Orondi in ten seconds, Lemmertz in less than two minutes, Diriks in 1 min. 32 sec., and Belling in less than twenty minutes, Jess Pedersen (of Denmark) in twenty minutes, and Van den Berg. I next engaged the German champion, Eberle, a very strong and accomplished wrestler, who gave up the struggle at the end of twenty minutes. This did not please the audience, and led to a scene of wild disorder. The police were called in and they put a stop to the whole tournament. There was nothing left for us but to start for home, which I accordingly did without having wrestled with Halil Adali.

Then on March 14, 1901, came a bolt from the blue in the shape of a telegram informing me that Dr Krajewski was dead. But a little time before I had seen the worthy doctor in the best of health, and I now learned that he had succumbed to apoplexy, after having been so unlucky as to fall and break a leg on the Fontanka Bridge on the Newski Prospekt. I, in common with all other Russian athletes, shed many a tear over the loss of this noble-hearted gentleman. In him I lost a friend who was almost a second father.

Towards the end of March another wrestling contest was held in St Petersburg. Amongst others I defeated the strong and nimble French wrestler, Lassartesse, in twenty minutes and Petroff in seven minutes, by an arm-roll or bras route, obtaining the first prize, a gold medal.

At Easter of this year (1901) the wrestling contest for the championship of the world began in Vienna. This championship I consider the biggest I ever gained, since never before nor since has such a wonderful array of contestants been gathered together. There were from Germany Jacobus Koch, H. Eberle, Stark, Axa, Missbach and Hitzler; from Belgium Omer de Bouillon and Clement le Terrassier; from Holland Dirk van den Berg; from Italy G. Raicevich, Figini; from Turkey Kara Ahmed, Halil Adali, and Coord Derelli; from Denmark Jess Pedersen; from America John Piening; from Austria Franzel, Sporer, Kreindl and Sprecht; from France Paul Pons, Laurent le Beaucairois, Aimable de la Calmette, and a whole host of lesser lights. Among others I defeated Omer de Bouillon, a most excellent Belgian wrestler, in nine minutes, and Hitzler in twelve minutes. It was here that the small but nimble Bayer caused such general astonishment by throwing the gigantic Turk, Halil Adali (who was 6 ft 2½ in. in height and weighed 20 st. 5 lb.) in a minute and a half, taking him by surprise with a brilliant bras route. I here made the acquaintance of a German wrestler named Koch, who was, I think, the best German wrestler I have ever seen. He was very strong and decidedly clever, but did not do much in Vienna on this occasion as he was not in particularly good form. I threw him in twenty minutes. I had heard a great deal of the American wrestler Piening and recently he sought notoriety in England by appearing against me. But he, too, though an excellent, if not particularly powerful wrestler, could do but little in Vienna. Pons, Adali, Laurent, and I were rather too good for him. Piening I threw in thirty-one seconds! Beaucairois fell in forty-one minutes, and Pons, in spite of a stubborn defence, in seventy-nine minutes. I had a pretty tough job with the tall Frenchman (6 ft 4½ in. in height and weighing over 18 st.), and my victory was greeted with generous applause. The Turk Halil Adali, whom I consider the best of all my opponents, was even stronger than Pons. Adali possessed gigantic strength and staying power, but I was in pretty good form and drew on the first day after wrestling for an hour and eighteen minutes. Next day, after a contest of forty minutes, the Turk gave in, being convinced that I must win. Indeed, I had wrestled in first-rate form, and had reduced the good man to a somewhat demoralised condition. The results came out as follows: Hackenschmidt, 1; Adali, 2; Pons, 3; etc.

From Vienna I went to Stettin, where I took first prize in a minor contest. In the middle of May a great wrestling contest was held in Berlin, and a number of excellent wrestlers were engaged, Lurich among others. There were two classes in this contest: Light-weights (85 kg. or 13 st. 5 lb. and under) and Heavy-weights (85 kg. or 13 st. 5 lb. and over). Consequently, on this occasion I did not meet Lurich, his weight at that time being 13 st. 4 lb. I was, however, somewhat astonished to find that on being matched against

Piening (whom I threw in thirty-one seconds in Vienna), he twice wrestled with him for an hour, the result being a draw in each case! I again threw Koch (in seven minutes), and several Berlin wrestlers in a few seconds, but in a contest with Pedersen, which I undertook by express desire of the management, I drew after a two hours' struggle. The whole contest was broken off owing to the failure of the management. The best wrestlers, including Petroff, Hitzler, Pohl, Pons, Pedersen, and myself, went on with the contest at the Metropole Theatre in Berlin. I now threw Hitzler in twenty-four, Petroff in thirty-one, and Pedersen in twenty-nine minutes. The German wrestler, Pohl, who finished second, and was left in the final heat with Pons and myself, was a new opponent to me. Pohl was very strong andclever. He threw Pedersen in three minutes. I defeated him in thirteen minutes, after an indecisive struggle of one hour on the previous evening. The periodical, Sport im Bild, commented on this match, in which it was generally thought that Pohl would prove a dangerous opponent, as follows:—" It was apparent from the very beginning of the final round (Hackenschmidt v. Pohl) that Hackenschmidt was in deadly earnest and anxious to bring matters to a crisis as soon as possible. Seizing Pohl round the body with irresistible force, he endeavored again and again to bring him to the ground, till at last he succeeded in doing so, though only at the cost of tremendous exertion. It then became clear that the Russian was resting for a moment and calling up a fresh reserve of strength, for he held Pohl motionless on the ground for some time. Then followed a sudden and violent ceinture de cote, from the left, to which Pohl nearly fell a victim. With one hand Hackenschmidt nearly jerked him on to his back. Then followed one or two remassements by means of which the Russian forced his opponent's head on to the ground, then another ceinture, which, however, failed to bring about the desired result. The struggle had lasted thirteen minutes, when Hackenschmidt at last secured the grip he so frequently employs with success. With his left hand he jerked Pohl so energetically that, in spite of his great weight (no kg. or 17 st. 4 lb.), the Hamburg champion fell fair and square on both shoulders. The whole character of the contest—in which Hackenschmidt attacked throughout, while Pohl remained on the defensive—proved conclusively that the Russian is greatly his superior in strength.

I wrestled with Pons, but at the end of the bout the Frenchman retired; after being twice within an ace of defeat, he was unable to continue owing to an accident to his arm. I was awarded first prize amid deafening applause, and received a gigantic laurel wreath, nearly 6 ft in diameter.

I spent a very pleasant time in Berlin and there made the acquaintance of the celebrated sculptor, Professor Reinhold Begas, who asked me to sit for him in the character of " Prometheus Vinctus." Professor Begas, a stately old man, who carried his seventy years well, took a great interest in wrestling, and was nearly always present during our contests.

I now returned home to rest and Went through several courses of treatment for the benefit of my arm, the most successful of these being the Priessnitsch cold-water pack. The measurement of my biceps, which had decreased to 15I in., rose again to 17½ in., and my weight went up from 14 st. 2 lb. to 15 st. 6 lb. After three months in October, 1901, I was able to take up wrestling again in Moscow. I was in excellent form, and, among other events, threw Lassartesse in seven minutes, Hitzler in twenty-one minutes, and the young Frenchman, Raoul le Boucher, a very powerful, young, heavy and skilful wrestler (6 ft 2½ in. in height and weighing. 19 st. 9 lb.), in twenty- three minutes in spite of a furious resistance on his part. I threw five excellent Moscow amateurs in seven minutes! This last tour de force I repeated shortly afterwards—at the end of October—in Munich, where I defeated five professional wrestlers also in seven minutes. After which. among others, I beat Burghardt (Austria) in six minutes, Cassino (France) in thirty seconds, Hitzler in twenty- three minutes, Rodel in twenty-seven seconds, Blatte (of Munich) in two and a half minutes, Eigemann (from Elberfeld) in less than one minute, Marchand (the Frenchman) in two minutes, and Koch in twenty-five minutes. I was next matched for the second time against the German champion, Eberle, who was now in better form than he had been at Hamburg. I was prepared for a fairly long struggle, in the event of his adopting defensive tactics, but to my surprise Eberle took the offensive against me. I gave him an opportunity of taking the lower hold from behind, and as I tightened this by a sturdy swing of the leg, I got him off his balance. He fell and I turned him quickly on his back. The whole contest, to the astonishment of every one, and especially of Eberle himself, only lasted five minutes.

On the following day, in company with the other wrestlers, I paid a visit to " Steierer Hans," a great character in Munich, who in his earlier days had travelled about the world in the role of Hercules, and had been unsurpassed in the lifting of weights with one finger. The worthy soul had now settled down to end his days in peace as an innkeeper. In an underground room he had a museum consisting chiefly of shapeless stones, axle- tons, and weights with which he performed various tricks for our benefit, accompanying them with amusing patter. Merely for the joke of the thing, I lifted with one hand a stone to which some weights were attached, the whole weighing 660 lb.

In November a small contest took place at Elberfeld, at which I was once more an easy winner.

On November 30, 1901, a contest for the wrestling championship of the world was commenced at the Casino de Paris. I had entered for this, and before it commenced, at an independent performance, I threw five professional wrestlers in six minutes altogether. For this tournament some hundred and thirty wrestlers had entered, and among others I defeated Mario in three and Buisson in three and three-quarter minutes. My first important adversary was Alexandre le Marseillais, a tall and heavy (17 st. 11 lb.) but none the less accomplished wrestler, whom I threw after a severe struggle of twenty minutes. I wrestled for one hour without result with Omer de Bouillon, who was in excellent form, but defeated him on the following day in twenty minutes.

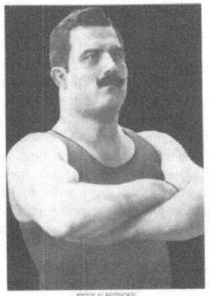

NICOLAI PETROFF
Hackenschmidt's Wrestling Tutor

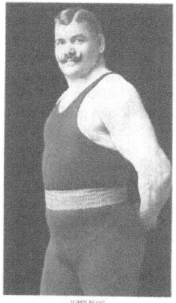

JOHN POHL

I now threw Koch in twenty minutes, Maurice Gambier in a short two minutes, Emile Vervet in six minutes, and the Frenchman, Raoul le Boucher, in twenty-one minutes.

Raoul wrestled somewhat savagely, but this did not avail him much, as I turned him with a " half-nelson," and got both his shoulders on the ground. At last my time came to wrestle with the celebrated Belgian, Constant le Boucher, in the final contest.

On this particular evening I happened to be in good form and as cool as ice. I got a splendid grip, and, to the general surprise of all, contrived to throw the Belgian after only eight minutes' wrestling. This was on December 19, 1901. I received a magnificent ovation, and the newspapers devoted whole columns of space to me.

On December 27 I wrestled once more with Constant, and was declared the winner after a long struggle. The final result of the tournament being as follows: First prize, of two gold medals and 3,000 frs, Hackenschmidt; one gold medal being awarded for having defeated all the four light-weight champions, and the other for beating the heavy weights. Second prize, a gold and a silver medal and 1,750 frs, Constant le Boucher. Third prize, with 700 frs, Omer de Bouillon. Fourth prize, and 450 frs, Raoul le Boucher. Fifth prize, and 300 frs, Hitzler. Sixth prize, and 200 frs, Emil Vervet; and so forth.

By the middle of January I felt it was high time for me to avail myself of an invitation to stay at Alsleben in Germany which I had received from Herr Siebert, the trainer, for my health had begun to suffer from my severe exertions during the championship contest. My weight had gone down to 14 st. 6 lb.

At Alsleben, which is a quiet little country town, I was able to give my nerves a thorough rest. The whole business of wrestling had become abhorrent to me. I had wrestled for a long time, without ceasing, hastening from one tournament to another.

I was tired of the arena, especially as my arm daily became more painful. I found in Siebert a man of the widest experience and soon conceived a liking for him. He strongly advised me to wait till I had fully recovered my health and taken a thorough rest before coming to any rash decision.

Thanks to quiet and good care, I throve amazingly, and very gradually commenced to train, under Siebert's guidance, with weights and dumbbells.

On January 27 I established a new world's record by raising a weight of 187 lb. behind my back with the knees bent. Not long after, for a wager, I jumped 100 times over a table with feet close together. In a word, my former depression gave place to the pleasures of life and vigour. I stayed a few weeks with Siebert, and during this time established the two following world's records:—

1. 110 lb. lifted fifty times with bent knees.
2. 90½ lb. in the right and 89½ lb. in the left hand held out simultaneously right and left at arm's length, but improved this afterwards to no and 100 lb. respectively.

About this time my patron, Count Ribeaupierre, wrote to me from St Petersburg suggesting that I should enter into an agreement with Herr Delmer, of Brussels, proprietor of the " Biceps." I had already an engagement with Herr Delmer, having consented to take part in a wrestling competition in Belgium, but had been prevented by ill-health from keeping my promise. I wrote to Herr Delmer. We soon came to an understanding, and now, restored to health and strength, I quitted Herr Siebert's hospitable roof, once more a wrestler heart and soul!

Early in the year 1902, I came over to England with the object of pitting myself against any opponent I could find.

For a long time this was not practicable, for just then the English public took but scant interest in wrestling, or, at any rate, in the Graeco-Roman branch of the Art, since few first-class exponents of this system had as yet visited Great Britain.

About this time an American wrestler named Carkeek made his appearance in London. I had known this man in France as an average wrestler. He was about forty years of age, and claimed, among other things, to have defeated Beaucairois, Gambier, and Pytlasinski. I sent more than one challenge to his manager, and also to Carkeek himself, but they were invariably refused. I was on the point of leaving England when it came to my knowledge that Carkeek, believing me to have already gone, had challenged any professional wrestler then in London to wrestle with him either in the Graeco-Roman, " Catch-as-catch-can," or Cornish styles, and would be sure to make a big advertisement out of my departure. I therefore purchased a box close to the stage (of the Alhambra), and as soon as Carkeek had finished his challenge, I sprang, accompanied by Mr Vansittart, the famous athlete, known as " The Man with the Grip of Iron," on to the stage in full wrestling costume, while my companion, holding a stake of £25 in his hand, challenged Carkeek to wrestle with me, and undertook to hand over the sum he held if I failed to throw Carkeek at least ten times within an hour. A tremendous uproar ensued, and, though the audience took our part, we were compelled to leave the stage by the police. On the following day I lodged £25 with the editor of the Sportsman on the conditions already announced from the stage. All the newspapers gave favorable notices of my debut, and on March 10 I received an engagement at the Tivoli Theatre, London. For some time my health suffered from a climate to which I was unaccustomed, but I nevertheless accepted further engagements, which were freely offered me.

In order to have a useful opponent for training purposes, I summoned my friend Koch from Germany, and we wrestled together almost every day for practice, wrestling continually for some months and defeating all opponents. Then I made the acquaintance of Tom Cannon, the well-known wrestler, who lives in Liverpool, and only wrestles occasionally now.

At the end of July Koch and I left England for the Continent and engaged in tournaments at Brussels, Liege, Namur and other places, in all of which I won the first prize, Koch generally succeeding in winning the second.

I then went back to England in order to wrestle a match with the renowned veteran, Tom Cannon. This took place on September 27, 1902, at Liverpool, and lasted thirty-three minutes. The English champion, though now somewhat of a veteran, had had a very wide and exceptionable experience, and was able to bring into play some very skilful, if somewhat painful, moves, which he had picked up from Turkish wrestlers. I managed, however, to secure a hammerlock and Cannon succumbed.

Not satisfied with this result, Cannon, after staying out a fifteen minute " limit," contest, made another match " to a finish " with me, which I won fairly easily.

This success, though not a very arduous one for me, was generally regarded as a great feather in my cap, and I received a number of excellent engagements to wrestle in England and Scotland in consequence.

I entered my name for the Gold Belt contest in Paris (November, 1902), but they sought to impose a number of peddling counter proposals, to which I could not see my way to consent, a result which seemed to be highly acceptable to the Paris authorities, as it was apparently intended that the favorite, Pons, whom I had already thrice defeated, should win. I did not regret this, as Pons is a first-rate man.

After this I toured all over England, being successful against every wrestler who accepted my challenge to all comers.

In 1903 I met and defeated the following wrestlers, Tom Cannon, Tom Connors, Tom MacInerney and Tom Clayton. I threw all of them, but was unfortunately laid up with an attack of rheumatism brought on by the damp climate of Glasgow, which prevented my taking part in the contest for the Championship of the World in Paris. In this contest Pedersen was first and Raoul le Boucher second, both of whom I had previously defeated.

Owing to the fact that the " Catch-as-catch-can " style of wrestling is the more usual and favourite method in England, I was frequently obliged to wrestle with my opponents in this method, but, thanks to my strength and presence of mind, I always came off the conqueror. I very often trained specially for this style with Jack Smith of Manchester, a very clever wrestler.

In September, 1903, I wrestled with Bech Olsen, who had, however, no claims to be considered a first-class wrestler. The contest however, came to an unsatisfactory termination, as, owing to an accident to my ankle, the match had to be discontinued.

On the strength of this, Antonio Pieri, " the terrible Greek," challenged me to wrestle with him, hoping that I would fall an easy victim. The match came off about the middle of October at the Oxford Music Hall, in London, and I threw this very experienced and—in spite of his years—very dangerous adversary, in twenty-five minutes. Pieri challenged me to a return match to be decided by one fall under Graeco-Roman, and one under " Catch-as- catch-can " rules. We met on November 21, and in the first bout (Graeco-Roman) I beat him in 17 min. 11 sec. by means of a " half-nelson," and in the second bout, which followed immediately after, in " Catch-as-catch- can " style, I threw him in 15 min. 25 sec.

Smarting under his defeat, Pieri set himself to work to unearth a wrestler who could beat me. And before very long he introduced to the British public a Turk named Ahmed Madrali, a man of gigantic strength, who was boomed in every possible manner, as being a better man than myself. At first I paid but little attention to these attacks, as I had a great many excellent engagements in London and in many other large English towns, where I defeated everyone who came into the ring against me. At last, however, I took up his challenge, and we met on January 30, 1904, at Olympia in London, the winning of two falls out of three to decide the match, the Turk being 6 ft 1 in. in height and weighing 16 st. A huge audience had assembled when the Turk entered the ring with Antonio Pieri, whilst I was accompanied by Koch. The contest, as will be remembered, was a very brief one, as on Madrali making a move for my waist, I dashed in and lifting him off his feet, threw him on to his shoulders. Unfortunately, he fell on his arm, and, as this was dislocated, he was unable to continue the contest, but luckily was able to begin wrestling again three months later.

This victory raised my reputation to its zenith, and since that time I do not think that I have had a wrestling rival in the affections or esteem of the British public.

There is no need for me to enter into any description of the troubles, legal and otherwise, connected with my next big encounter. They were far from being pleasant to either Jenkins or myself, but since neither of us wished to disappoint the public, we readily agreed to the final makeshift arrangements and met on the mat before 6,000 people at the Albert Hall on July 2,1904. I early on succeeded in getting " behind " the American champion, but after a five minutes' struggle he succeeded in breaking loose. Three times afterwards I threw him on the mat, but he managed to wriggle out of a fall. Jenkins struggled hard and displayed very good defensive tactics, but was forced finally to succumb to a " half-nelson " after 20 min. 37 sec. wrestling. After fifteen minutes' interval Jenkins opened the second bout with an aggressive movement, and for some little time we had a stand-up struggle. Again we went to the mat, where, in spite of his utmost efforts, I finally managed to pin him out after 14 min. 27 sec.

The Sportsman report of this match read as follows:

" It was ten o'clock before the rivals appeared on the platform. By this time the spectators were in a high state of enthusiasm and gave the men a ringing cheer. Taking stock of the two men it was clear that Hackenschmidt had the advantage, physically speaking, at every turn. He looked a stone and a half heavier, deeper and more solid about the chest, more firmly set on the limbs, and to have nearly twice the muscular development of the American. Jenkins is a strongly-built man, but he did not appear half so fit as his opponent, carrying too much flesh. For all that, he made a creditable show, and gave one the impression of being a man of real grit, resource and stamina.

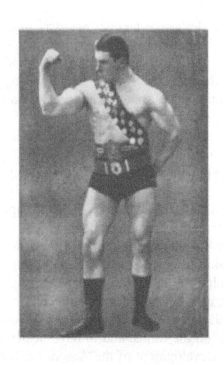

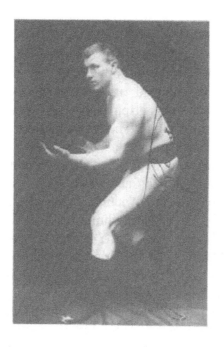

" When the men got to grips, Hackenschmidt attacked in decisive style, and twice just missed with the flying mare. In less than three minutes he fixed his rival in a cruel body grip and swung him over on to the stage. Jenkins endeavored to spring forward on to his feet, but Hackenschmidt's arms shot out like lightning, and he pulled his man down with the greatest ease. The American defended very cleverly, and, failing to find an opening for an arm-hold, the Russian picked his opponent up with the intention of pitching him over his back. Jenkins smartly eluded his grip, and after six minutes both were on their feet. Hackenschmidt was forcing the pace at a terrific rate, and three times lifted his man up and brought him to the boards with a magnificent display of strength, but it availed nothing against the American's skilful defence. Again Hackenschmidt attempted the flying mare, but his hand slipped on his opponent's neck, and like a flash Jenkins gripped the Russian by the waist and had him down. The wrestling was now more even, and each man attacked in turn. The strength and science which the challenger exhibited were a complete revelation, and he kept his opponent at bay without much difficulty. When a quarter of an hour had gone, Hackenschmidt rushed in and swung Jenkins bodily round the stage, describing three circles before he threw him to the boards, but the American once more eluded his grip like an eel. Then the Russian braced himself for a big effort. Twice he twisted Jenkins over on to one shoulder, and just as promptly did Jenkins, with a mighty contraction of his neck and shoulder muscles, snap the holds. At this point Jenkins mysteriously weakened. Hackenschmidt bore down on him with the power of a Hercules, and with a pedal action similar to a man pushing a heavy roller up a hill, forced his man over on his back, and with an irresistible ' half-nelson' gained the first fall in 20 min. 37 sec.

" In the second bout Hackenschmidt did most of the attacking, but Jenkins again put up a wonderfully plucky and skilful defence. Once the latter forgot himself and the rules by employing the leg-hold, but Hackenschmidtappeared quite unruffled by an act which ought to have been penalized by disqualification. Minute after minute sped by, but Jenkins could put on nothing more dangerous than a back-of-the-neck hold in answer to the Russian's arm-hold. Then Hackenschmidt brought the ' half-nelson' into play, but when Jenkins seemed in hopeless plight he extricated himself by a magnificent feat of wrestling, subtlety that evoked a tremendous storm of cheering. It proved his last expiring effort, however, for before he had quite recovered from the exhaustion which the struggle had engendered, the Russian had cleverly slipped on a second ' half-nelson,' and Jenkins was placed squarely on his shoulders in 14 min. 27 sec. Jenkins is to be congratulated on his plucky fight and his fine display of wrestling. The cheer which he received after his defeat was quite as hearty as that accorded Hackenschmidt."

Leaving England in September, 1904, I set out for a four months' tour in the Antipodes. My first experiences of Australia were unfortunately by no means as pleasant as they might have been, for I had to go into hospital very soon after my arrival in Sydney. I was not able to fulfill any of my engagements for quite five weeks, owing to both my arm and my knee again giving way. I was suffering from what are commonly called a housemaid's knee and a miner's elbow, which means water on both joints, necessitating an operation.

This was successful, and I was able to get to work, touring through all the principal towns and meeting all the wrestlers of note whom I could come across. Prior to my arrival in the Southern Continent, the two wrestlers who had enjoyed the biggest reputations were two big Hindus, Buttan Singh and Gunga Brahm. Both of these were fine big men, with plenty of strength and considerable skill, yet I threw the pair of them in nine minutes on the same night.

Clarence Weber, however, the Champion All-round Athlete of Australia, a most splendidly built young fellow, managed to hold out for ten minutes on more than one occasion. I may say, though, that I did not make any special preparation for either of these encounters, and owing, of course, to my having to wrestle different opponents nearly every night, I was naturally a bit weary and lacking in fire and vigour.

As Graeco-Roman wrestling was not well understood in Australia, I found it occasionally difficult to fix up matters with the various opponents who presented themselves and was in consequence compelled to devote my attention seriously to the study of the " Catch-as-catch-can " style. This was an important stage in my career and, considering that I was practically staking all my hard-earned reputation on my prospects of success under these new and comparatively strange rules, a somewhat risky step to contemplate. Nevertheless I accepted the situation, and can sincerely acknowledge that I have never regretted having done so.

After a fairly considerable experience, I may now confess that I distinctly prefer the more open method, and do not again propose deserting catch-as-catch-can. I have indeed made publicly a declaration of my determination never to wrestle under Graeco-Roman rules again.

By the way, on one occasion while in Australia, I was challenged to wrestle in the Cornish style of wrestling, in which a fall is secured only when a wrestler is thrown on any three points, viz., both shoulders and one hip, or both hips and a shoulder touch the ground. All bouts are contested from a standing position, and a hold is secured on the jacket which each contestant has to wear.

My challenger, Delhi Nielsen, who was an experienced Cornish wrestler, may perhaps have imagined that at this style (to which I was quite unaccustomed) he might very probably enjoy a comparatively even chance with me. He having defeated over 400 opponents and possessing an untarnished record was, in fact, very confident.

He consequently refused to wrestle me, save under these conditions, and I was compelled to agree to his terms, trusting that my acquaintance with the Russian style of wrestling, with waist-belts (between which and the Cornish style there is a very faint resemblance, although tripping is prohibited under the Russian rules), might stand me in good stead.

Be that as it may, I was able to rise to the occasion and to throw him very easily.

Having completed my Australian engagements, during the course of which I defeated Grotz, who was called the Champion of South Africa, and several other prominent wrestlers and physical culturists, I paid a brief visit to New Zealand, and then sailed for America, where I was booked for several engagements, the most important of all being my return match with Tom Jenkins, the American champion, whom I had defeated under Graeco-Roman rules at the Albert Hall on July 2, 1904.

On my way across the Pacific, I made a brief stay at the island of Samoa, and can well understand the enthusiasm with which travelers in the South Seas always refer to those havens of bliss, the islands of Polynesia.

I had promised to meet Jenkins in this return encounter in New York, after the London contest, and now agreed that our second meeting should be under Catch-as-catch-can " rules, with which my opponent was more familiar, but at which style I had but little experience, save for an occasional encounter in England and more frequently during my Australian tour.

This match with Jenkins, however, was the first big one in which I had engaged entirely under "Catch-as- catch-can " rules, and considerable interest was, perhaps, naturally felt throughout America on this account.

Jenkins and I met before a huge crowd at the Madison Square Gardens, New York, on May 4, 1905, our respective weights being as follows: Jenkins 14 st. 4 lb. and my own 14 st. 12 lb.

I was not yet sufficiently versed in the style at which we were wrestling to forestall the clever leg-locks and holds by which my opponent contrived to postpone disaster. He was mostly on the defensive, wriggling and extricating himself from difficulties in a very able manner, but despite a very strenuous struggle and a determined bridge, I finally managed to lever him over and pin him down in 31 min. 15 sec.

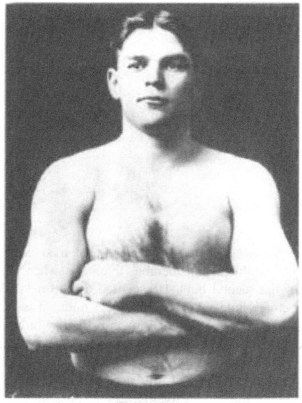

FRANK GOTCH

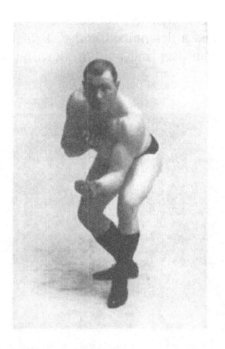

He seemed very exhausted, but recovered well, and exhibited considerable liveliness when we met for the second bout. He secured a "half-nelson" and a crotch-hold, and several times initiated an attack, but I did not experience much difficulty in breaking clear from the holds he managed to secure. I gradually wore him down, and, finally fixing a "half-nelson," forced him over despite his struggles, pinning him down for the second time in 22 min. 4 sec.

A typical American report of this match ran as follows:

New York, May 5.—Geo. Hackenschmidt, the Russian Lion, defeated Tom Jenkins, the American champion wrestler, in two straight falls last night at

Madison Square garden, in a match in which Jenkins was handled like a pigmy in the hands of a giant, Hackenschmidt broke holds as if they were the clutchings of a child.

For half an hour the Russian Lion battered Jenkins without a moment's cessation. The older man's vitality began to ebb. Suddenly Hackenschmidt got an " half- nelson " lock on him—both hands up under the chest and clasped around his neck. Inch by inch he twisted Jenkins over, still over, till both shoulders touched the mat. But Referee Hurst did not see the fall and signaled to go on. Within a minute Hackenschmidt repeated the feat, and this time he kept his man bored down until Hurst dragged him off. Time, 31 min. 15 sec.

Tom was still tired when he came back fifteen minutes later for the second bout. Patiently, bravely, unflinchingly, almost hopefully, he put forth all his cunning and strength. Once, as they stood face to face, Hackenschmidt seized Jenkins under the arms and whirled him around in a furious waltz. The body of Jenkins stood out straight, his feet pointing at the horizon. Twice thus around he went; then Hackenschmidt slammed him down on the floor. Tom wriggled around so that his shoulders did not touch the mat. It was a wonderful exhibition of quick thinking under adverse circumstances. But Tom's bolt was shot. No mere human giant could last under the awful strain ofhandling Hackenschmidt. After 22 min. and 4 sec. the Russian again put Jenkins down with a "half- nelson." Poor old Tom was hardly able to walk out of the ring. Hackenschmidt dashed away as briskly as ever.

" I would like to have thrown him quicker," he said, " but several times when I had good holds on him he turned very white and I was afraid of hurting him, so I let up."

Despite the strenuous nature of this match, I felt very little fatigue or exhaustion afterwards, thanks to my excellent condition. I was able to demonstrate this on the following evening, when I was matched to throw half-a- dozen wrestlers of considerable local prominence under Graeco-Roman rules. This was a fairly stiff contract, but I managed to dispose of the whole half-dozen inside eighteen minutes.

James Parr, the old Lancashire wrestler, then challenged me to throw him the next evening, offering to resist being thrown three times within the hour. He was, of course, giving a fair amount of weight, but as he is a very skilful wrestler I consider that I did not do at all badly by pinning him down three times in 7 min. 50 sec.

During my tour in the States I had a rather amusing experience in St Louis. I was there matched against Jean Baptiste, who was the champion wrestler of the district.

As soon as the match was arranged I was attacked by malarial fever, and, consulting a doctor, was ordered to bed, where I speedily became much worse, my temperature rising as high as 105 degrees.

Under these circumstances, and especially as the doctor considered my condition to be highly critical, I sent to the match promoters and informed them that it would be impossible for me to fulfill my engagement on the date agreed.

They called to see me in a state of great distress, represented that their outlay had been considerable, that they had sold a large number of tickets, and that if they were forced to return the money they had received for these they would be completely ruined.

They implored me to meet Baptiste and used so many arguments that I was practically compelled to assent, provided I found myself able to leave my bed, and although I was still very ill on the day of the match I managed to struggle down to the scene of our encounter.

Arrived there with the doctor by my side, I felt so weak, ill and giddy, that I could not summon up sufficient energy to change my attire, and was sitting shivering and shaking with fever, when I overheard my opponent in the next dressing-room asserting that he would not meet me, as I should be sure to kill him. The promoters were busy trying to encourage him, and as a last resource brought him into my dressing-room that I might assure him that I would be gentle and would handle him tenderly.

I was able to do this confidently, as at the moment I felt scarcely strong enough to wrestle with a child.

However, the humor of the situation so appealed to me that I had difficulty in restraining my laughter, and after Baptiste, now somewhat more courageous, had retired to get ready I was able to undress and to get into my wrestling trunks.

I felt somewhat better, but was still so weak that I positively reeled as I mounted the steps to the raised platform on which we were to wrestle, and experienced considerable difficulty in getting through the ropes which surrounded the mat.

Once there, my strength seemed to come back to me, and the sight of my timid adversary nerved me to go through the ordeal.

In his state of nervousness and terror, he was, perhaps, not a very formidable opponent, but he was, nevertheless, very big and strong and but for the nervous strength with which I have been endowed and which seemed to suddenly come back to me in full tide, I might have had a stiff bargain.

However, as matters went, I did not experience much trouble, throwing him three times in fairly quick time, and subsequently a Turk, Ali Muralah by name. This last opponent was styled " the terrible Turk," but I had never heard of him before that day, nor have I heard of him since. After which I returned to bed and to my doctor's care and indignation. He was very wroth and told me that I had practically done my best to commit suicide, but my constitution pulled me through, and I have since experienced no ill effects from my adventure.

After finishing my engagements in the States I paid a visit to Canada, where I threw such opponents as I could meet with. The most formidable of these was the celebrated French-Canadian, Emile Maupas, a strong and clever wrestler. He is an adept at the reversed body hold, which he tried on with me, but barely succeeded in lifting me from the mat, then losing his balance and falling backwards. I threw him three times in less than twenty- one and a half minutes, the first fall occupying 7 min. 39 sec., the second 6 min. 19 sec., and the third 7 min. 20 sec.

After visiting the Falls of Niagara, and doing a little sightseeing, I again set sail for England, where I was booked to appear for a week in Manchester, before appearing at the Canterbury Music Hall on Whit- Monday.

Back again in the British Isles with a long list of music-hall engagements before me and having anticipations of a prospective match with Alexander Munro (the Scottish champion) and a possible return encounter with Madrali, it was quite clear that on these occasions my opponents would stipulate for " Catch-as-catch-can " conditions, and that it would be advisable for me to accustom myself thoroughly to that style of wrestling.

I therefore resolved that, at all events for the time being, I would only engage in contests or exhibitions under that code, more especially as there can be no doubt of its greater popularity among the British people. Several months elapsed before the conditions could be arranged for my encounter with Munro, and meanwhile I had my music-hall engagements to fulfill, but finally, on October 28, 1905, I encountered the British champion before 16,000 spectators on the Glasgow Rangers' Football Ground, at Ibrox Park. The greatest interest was evinced in the encounter on account of my antagonist's magnificent physique and great reputation. My readers may, perhaps, be interested in comparing our respective weights and measurements on that occasion:—

	MUNRO	HACKENSCHMIDT
Height	6 ft.	5 ft. 9½ in.
Weight	15 st. 5 lb.	14 st. 8 lb.
Neck	18½ in.	22 in.
Chest	48 in.	52 in.
Waist	36 in.	34 in.
Thigh	27 in.	26¾ in.
Calf	17 in.	18 in.
Forearm	14½ in.	15½ in.
Biceps	17¾ in.	19 in.

A drizzling rain which fell throughout the contest somewhat hampered my movements, and since I was the attacking party during most of the time the conditions naturally handicapped me more seriously than my adversary. Munro was the first to go to the mat, and was soon compelled to " bridge " for safety. I turned him over with a leg hold, but he managed to slip clear, as he also did out of several " half-nelsons." Indeed, after about a quarter of an hour's struggle he managed so to extricate himself from my grasp as to be able to put in several aggressive movements. He was, and is undoubtedly, a very powerful man, and did not finally succumb (to a "half- nelson") until after a struggle lasting altogether 22 min. 40 sec.

After ten minutes' interval we commenced the second bout, and again the Scotchman displayed fine defensive tactics, once or twice even assuming the offensive. Again, however, I got him with a " half-nelson " and rolled him over in 11 min. 11 sec.

That night, on appearing to fulfill my engagement at the Palace Theatre, just outside Glasgow, the audience called for a speech, and after my saying a few words they stood up as one man and gave me one of the biggest ovations I had ever experienced in Great Britain. The kindly enthusiasm with which they acclaimed me as "a jolly good fellow" was such as I shall never forget, for the rest of my life.

My music-hall engagements, together with an occasional brief holiday, occupied me now for the next six months, when, in order to satisfy Madrali, Pieri, the British public and myself that the result of our first encounter was not, as Pieri alleged, " a fluke," I consented to again meet the " Terrible Turk " under " Catch-as-catch-can " rules on this occasion. At this style of wrestling he was, according to his mentor and discoverer, " absolutely invincible," and on the strength of recent encounters with Tom Jenkins and Alex. Munro, a not inconsiderable section of the public inclined to the opinion that he would " make me travel." Even I myself had but little confidence in my chance, consequently I trained seriously for the occasion, putting in a fortnight's preparation at dear old Jack Crumley's house, " The Seven Stars," Shepherd's Bush. I had practice bouts regularly with one or other of the following very capable group of wrestlers: Jack Smith, " Gunner " Moir, poor Jack Grumley, John Strong, Gus Rennart, and Constables Barrett and Humphreys of the City Police, and to wind up, I took them all to Worthing and finished my training there.

One daily item of my training may deserve mention here, since in itself it was no small feat and graduated according to circumstances might be included with advantage in every wrestler's preparation. I used to kneel down while the others placed a sack of cement weighing six hundredweight on my back, and as soon as this was comfortably settled, poor Jack Grumley, who scaled another 232 lbs, seated himself thereon, say, well over 900 lbs in all. No small weight-moving feat I can assure you.

Under these circumstances, therefore, it can be well understood that I was feeling particularly fit and well when for the second occasion I faced Madrali at Olympia.

As this contest was brought about after a tremendously wordy discussion in the Press and amidst the greatest possible excitement, it may, perhaps, interest my readers if I quote the report which appeared in The Manchester Guardian, which runs as follows:—

" Hackenschmidt and Madrali, surrounded by their friends and seconds, were early in their dressing-rooms. Madrali was reported marvelously fit, but a whisper flew around, among the journalists, telling the alarming tale that Hackenschmidt was sick! His stomach was wrong! They were anointing him with alcohol! He was faint! He was trembling! Part of it was true. Sheer excitement had upset the Russian, and betting began to veer, and the odds weakened just as they do on the morning of a big race, when the favorite is reported to be coughing. Strung to a higher pitch of excitement by this ' stable intelligence,' the crowd watched and waited hungrily for the appearance of the two mighty men. It was nearly half-past nine before the band played with great gusto, ' See the conquering hero comes ! ' There was a sudden eddy among the group of privileged persons at the side of the ring, the eddy broke and through it strode Madrali. Olympia howled as one man. The Turk stalked on to the stage like a ghost in a dream. He looked immense—passionless and colorless; a black overcoat covered him from throat to ankles. . . . He walked to his corner as an automaton walks and sat down stiffly on a kitchen chair. At the tail end of the cheers which greeted him came Hackenschmidt, in a brown dressing-gown, with tassels flapping dolorously. With his wonderful shoulders concealed by the wrappings of his gown, he appeared small and puny compared with the great mass of humanity opposite him. His face— frank and boyish as a rule— was the very picture of misery. It was drab and drawn and withered. His lips were trembling and his eyes were flashing furtive glances across the great auditorium, whilst the cheers hurtled among the rafters of the glass dome

"At the call of time,' and in a silence through which one little cough broke like a rifle shot, the Turk and the Russian leaped like cats to the mat. And at that moment life and confidence came back to Hackenschmidt, whose apparent collapse was nothing more than tremendous excitement worked up to a pitch almost heartbreaking. He knew that in the " Catch-as-catch-can " style Madrali was cunning and relentless if he could only get time— time to wear his man down and to grind the spirit out of him. And Hackenschmidt's one idea was to limit the time to a mere handful of seconds, if he only could, and not save himself for an endurance test. After a few lightning flashes of preliminary sparring the Russian jumped in for a neck hold and got Madrali's head down. But Madrali weaved his arms around Hackenschmidt's waist and hugged and tugged until his opponent bent nearly double. Hackenschmidt made a wild grab at the Turk's neck and got a hold which was near enough to the " strangle grip " to cause Madrali to squirm away and protest, mumbling to the referee as he explained in pantomimic passes with his hands. In another moment the pair were at it again, crouching like tigers for a spring. And here Madrali made his first bad mistake. He tried his favorite dodge—a sudden spring to get a leg hold. But Hackenschmidt, sharp as a needle, was on the look-out for that. He hopped back an inch and no more, Madrali's hand smote the air and the impetus of his fruitless grab upset his balance. His right arm went up to steady himself, and like an arrow, the Russian leaped in, took his man under that right arm and swung him round. Down with a thud and a grunt went the Turk. Hackenschmidt was on him, and Madrali went over in a body-roll, which no power on earth could stop. There was one wild struggle, a helpless kick or two, and Madrali was pinned to the carpet in a fair and straight throw in 1 min. 34 sec. Madrali staggered up, shook himself, and stalked back to his corner, while in a storm of cheers Hackenschmidt, pale as death but smiling, slipped on his dressing-gown and departed to his dressing-room for the fifteen

minutes' interval. Madrali stayed where he was, solacing himself with a rough towel.
" For the second bout the Russian was a raging favorite. And lo! in the second bout Madrali found his haven. Twice he dived for the leg hold. Twice he got it, being craftier this time, after his first stinging lesson in carelessness. Twice Hackenschmidt broke away. And then in a whirl of heaving flesh both men came to earth with a bump. Madrali was on top. He wriggled behind the Russian and wrapped his sinewy arms round his waist. Hackenschmidt crouched on all fours, while Madrali kneaded him remorselessly—a painful process which has churned many a great wrestler into sickness and partial unconsciousness. A minute or so of this set the Russian sweating. His white skin glistened in the blaze of the electric light. His face was twisted with pain. And still the inexorable Turk gruelled and gruelled his opponent. Thinking, no doubt, he had weakened him sufficiently, he made a grab at his ankle. That did not come off, so Madrali ground his knee into the Russian's thigh. This was not strictly cricket, and Mr Dunning promptly stopped it. Hackenschmidt just watched for his chance. It came with startling suddenness. Incautiously Madrali loosed his waist hold and tried a "half- nelson " on the Russian's right arm, but found it too strong even for his muscles, whereupon Hackenschmidt got a left wrist hold and a leg-lock simultaneously, strained the mighty muscles of his shoulders almost to bursting- point and with a heave which showed incredible strength hurled his man clean over. The crowd went mad with excitement. '

He's got him! He's got him!' they yelled. He had. Fiercely, furiously, panting and straining Hackenschmidt flung his whole weight upon the prostrate Turk. It was the biggest effort he had ever made. For a breathless moment Madrali struggled. Then he collapsed with a sob, and Mr Dunning smote Hackenschmidt upon the shoulders with a sounding slap which signalized that the championship had been won and that the terrible Turk had been beaten. ' Time, four minutes,' cried Mr Mansell, the timekeeper, and like an avalanche, the crowd swarmed, roaring into the arena."

Since that date it has become fashionable in certain quarters to call Madrali a much overrated man. There never was a worse, or indeed a more absurd, mistake. He was a most formidable opponent, one of the strongest, if not actually the strongest, man I have ever encountered. Somewhat careless, perhaps, as a wrestler, but once he had you in his clutches—well, he had me pretty tightly, I admit, and I was able to turn the tables, but I shall always count myself as singularly fortunate in having been able to do so. Tom Jenkins is a very powerful man and a most able wrestler, and yet Madrali positively crushed him. Munro is one of the strongest men in the world, and thoroughly experienced at "Catch-as-catch-can" and yet Madrali treated him almost as if he were a novice. No, the opinions which were entertained of the " terrible Turk " prior to his defeat by me were much nearer the truth than those which obtained subsequently thereto, and every wrestler who ever felt Madrali's grip will, I am sure, fully endorse this opinion.

I was now booked up for a lengthy tour, during which I visited nearly every town in the United Kingdom, meeting all the wrestlers of repute in every locality, without coming across any serious or exciting encounter.

In August, 1907, my old knee trouble again made its appearance, but this time the water gathered in the joint itself, so that my knee cap stood away from the joint quite a quarter of an inch. By medical advice I now always wore a bandage, and found it practically impossible to do any serious wrestling practice. Even a slow trot caused me such pain that I could only fulfill my ordinary engagements with the utmost difficulty.

Matters in the Wrestling World were livened up however by the visit of three wrestlers possessing formidable reputations on the Continent.

First came Constant le Marin, then the Galician wrestler Cyganiewicz, or Zbysco. Finally came the big Cossack Padoubny, the winner of World's Championship Tournaments in the Graeco-Roman style.

These were followed by Joe Rogers, a big American wrestler, with whom I had wrestled in New York, but who had since progressed considerably in his knowledge of the game.

All four of these hurled challenges at me, but as I found that Constant le Marin, who had been first in the field, appeared less ready to come to business than he had been to announce his readiness therefor, and as it would have been absurd to match myself to meet them all at once or to lay myself open to their accusations, if I accorded either of them precedence, I suggested that they had better wrestle among themselves, promising to meet the winner.

Knowing full well that they were all formidable opponents, and feeling the urgent need of rest and recuperation after my long and arduous spell of work, I now took a brief holiday, paying a visit to my home in Russia.

Unfortunately I did not find the rest or cure I needed, and consequently returned to England feeling far from fit and well, in time to witness the Zbysco-Padoubny match, to which the proposed tournament had dwindled down.

This, as you are probably aware, resulted in the victory of Zbysco, owing to the disqualification of Padoubny, and I accordingly signed articles to meet the winner.

Meanwhile Rogers, who had been unable to enter the proposed tournament or triangular contest, owing to a poisoned thumb, was clamoring for a match with me, on the plea that I had promised to meet him while I was in America, if he took up wrestling seriously and was able to prove that he was a serious opponent.

This he had done by virtue of his success in one or two American tournaments in which he had defeated some very formidable opponents and so I consented to meet him.

We came together at the Oxford Music Hall on February 6, 1908, and, despite his great advantage in height and weight (he is quite six inches taller and more than three stone heavier than I was), I did not experience any very great difficulty in pinning him out twice in 7 min. 35 sec. and 6 min. 45 sec. respectively.

I was attacking practically throughout the contest, almost the only aggressive move which he made being an attempt to seize me round the thighs, which resulted in his being thrown for the first time, as I stooped also and quicker than he did, securing a hold just below his knees, lifting him and then pitching him forcibly to the ground, after which I was able to pin him down without much difficulty.

I then sailed to America to fulfill my contract to wrestle Frank Gotch. Prior to the contest itself I fulfilled a night's engagement at the Grand Central Palace, New York, meeting Neil Olsen, a quick little wrestler, who calls himself Young Hackenschmidt, and Steg-Miller, whom I took with me to America. After this I went to Boston, where I wrestled John Perelli, Albert Ouvray and several others; and had the honor of making the acquaintance of the son of President Roosevelt, who introduced me to his friends. From Boston I went to Philadelphia, and there beat Carl Darschn of Camden, in 3| min., Henry Paulson in 5 min. 9 sec., and Miller. From Philadelphia I went to Washington, where I was introduced to President Roosevelt at the White House, and to several other leading politicians. There I wrestled five opponents, and threw them all pretty quickly; travelling thence to Baltimore, where, after defeating two or three opponents, I wrestled 15 min. with Gus Schonlein (America). From here I went straight to Chicago to get ready for Gotch.

As to the contest itself so much has been said and written already by various eyewitnesses and also by people who were not eyewitnesses, that it seems to me that I should be serving no useful purpose by either adding to or taking from the remarks I have already made on the subject.

After returning to England I had to prepare for a match with Zbysco, which should have taken place in June. I started hard practice, but in a short time felt such pain in my right knee, round the knee cap, that it was even painful to walk. Any quick turn made me feel as though I should collapse. I cancelled all my engagements, including the match, and went to Aix-la-Chapelle, to undergo a thorough treatment. Examination by one of the leading surgeons proved the necessity for an immediate serious operation, from which I am now recovering.

I have been asked whether I propose seeking to regain my lost championship.

Well, in order to answer that question, I beg to state that the only man I propose wrestling before my final retirement is Frank Gotch, and then to inquire as to the championship which I am alleged to have lost.

When did I last hold one?

When I entered for and won the Championship Tournaments in Vienna, Berlin and Paris in the year 1901, the motive that actuated me was the desire to prove myself a greater wrestler than all the famous exponents of the science who were gathered together at those places. That I won the title of champion at the same time was purely a side issue.

So much so, indeed, that I have not since troubled about renewing it.

Throughout my whole career I have never bothered as to whether I was a champion or not a champion. The only title I have desired to be known by is simply my name, George Hackenschmidt.

Made in the USA
Las Vegas, NV
06 December 2024